D0107126

ART
OF THE
INNER MEAL

The Power of Mindful Practices

to Heal Our Food Cravings

Donald Altman

moon lake media

New Revised Edition

First Paperback Printing 2002

A hardcover edition of this book was published in 1999 by HarperSanFrancisco

Cover Design by Bruce Hanson, Ramsden Fine Arts. Illustrations by Paul Mendoza.

While the author and publisher have done everything possible to include information from many religions and
disciplines, we assume no liability or responsibility for inaccuracies, errors, omissions, and inconsistencies
rendered in the creation of this book. Any slights of people or organizations are fully unintentional. When
deciding upon food-related practices or diets, readers must use their own best judgment and should consult
with doctors and nutritionists if necessary.

Publisher's Cataloging-in-Publication

(Provided by Quality Books, Inc.)

Altman, Don, 1950–
    Art of the inner meal : the power of mindful
practices to heal our food cravings / Donald Altman. --
Rev., 1st pbk. ed.
    p. cm.
    Includes bibliographical references and index.
    ISBN 0-9639161-3-0

    1. Food--Religious aspects. 2. Religions.
3. Spiritual life. I. Title.

BL65.F65A485 2002   291.4'46
                            QBI02-200703

Acknowledgments:

My heartfelt thanks and appreciation to all who gave so generously of their time and knowledge. In particular—Venerable U Silananda; Brother Brahmananda and Lauren Landress of the Self-Realization Fellowship; Rabbi Don Singer; U Thondara, Ashin U Thitzana, the monks and community of the Burma Buddhist Monastery; Roy Parker, O.H.C. and the brothers of Mount Calvary Monastery; Dr. Ahmad H. Sakr of the Islamic Education Center; Tea Master Tomiko Numano.

Thanks, also, to Randy and Jim—as well as others—who shared valuable ideas, feedback, and supported my efforts in ways too numerous to mention. Special loving thanks to my mother Barbara and to the love of my life, Sanda.

May all beings be blessed with peace,
compassion, and loving-kindness.

Contents

Part One
SPIRITUAL INGREDIENTS

Introduction

Part Two
OUR MINDFUL SEASONINGS

Part Three
RETURN TO SOURCE

Part One

SPIRITUAL INGREDIENTS

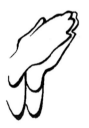

Introduction

There are few things in life more capable of filling us with joy and pleasure on a daily basis than food and eating. The memories of food may even go back to our first years, shaping our tastes, our desires, and even our emotional needs. But learning to live in peace with food is not so easy. Temptation is always present, always lurking. How can we, both figuratively and literally, avoid stumbling from cheesecake to cheesecake? How can we embrace food in a balanced, healthy way that nourishes mind, body, and spirit?

The struggle with food is universal. It abounds in our history, myth, and wisdom traditions. How ironic that so many of us should suffer physically and emotionally from what is intended to be the most basic and nourishing of actions. Why has something as healing as food become so problematic in modern life? Can we ever hope to regain a sense of balance and harmony? I believe so, which is why creating a new, healing relationship with food is what this book is about.

All things, it seems, follow a journey of sorts—even books. This revised and expanded paperback edition of *Art of the Inner Meal* adds the benefit of my experiences leading Mindful Eating workshops and retreats. Can mindfulness really change how we relate to food? Recently, the practice of mindfulness has been validated in some treatment programs for those with eating problems. One successful program combines the practice of mindfulness with a cognitive behavior therapy known as Dialectical Behavior Therapy, or DBT. Eating problems can be difficult to treat. Modern interest in the healing capabilities of ancient mindfulness gives hope to all who struggle with food cravings.

Shortly after *Art of the Inner Meal* was first published, I was invited to appear as a guest on a syndicated radio program hosted by a talk-show psychologist. She began the segment by disclosing that she had come to the conclusion that a spiritual component was necessary for healing eating problems. Of course, I didn't argue the point! I have witnessed firsthand how mindful practices can alter our perception in powerful and enduring ways.

This revised paperback edition differs slightly in emphasis from the hardcover. Naturally, it includes all the same spiritual and mindful practices. Drawn from various traditions, these techniques hold the potential to lessen food cravings and give us more freedom of choice. In addition, the paperback focuses more on practical tools by including several unique exercises developed in the workshop setting. As well, it ties all the pieces together with an all-new chapter on the essential "Six Steps to Changing Food Habits."

If you are spiritually oriented, you can view this book and its methods as spiritual. If not, you can simply use mindfulness and other tools as a way to attain deeper awareness. Either way, this path offers freedom from our desires and a new relationship with the present moment. Such is the journey of the *inner meal.*

1 - Beginnings...

CHEF PRIMO
(raises food to her mouth)
Now taste. Taste it.

ANN
(she tastes)
Oh my God... Oh my God.

CHEF PRIMO
You like?

ANN
Oh my God!

CHEF PRIMO
*"Oh my God" is right. See? Now you know—
to eat good food is to be close to God.*

— from the film, *Big Night*

As a boy growing up in Chicago, I found Sunday to be one of the most happily anticipated days of the week. For this was the day I spent visiting and eating with my cousins at the apartment of my *bubby* and *zadie*—the Yiddish words for "grandmother" and "grandfather." I still remember how everyone inspected the kitchen like Sherlock Holmes, hoping to find a scent of our grandmother's spectacular homemade apple pie. Soon, all the family members scurried to the table to take their familiar seats.

The air weighed heavily from the smell of rich, pungent European food—gefilte fish, latkes, and matzo ball soup—exotic dishes that I never got to eat at home. Bread and wine were blessed with prayer. The bittersweet, dark red wine always made my mouth pucker and face convulse. Strange Yiddish words I'd never heard before were spoken; I felt certain this was an adult plot to keep the best jokes from the tender ears of us youngsters. Stories and laughter came one after another in nonstop waves.

The whole dynamic of my immediate family shifted, too. My father, often pained by migraines and easily provoked, mellowed out considerably to show a side of himself that was more carefree, forgiving, and composed. During this special Sunday meal, differences melted away and everyone was accepted, no questions asked. The only purpose was to be with family, be comfortable, and have fun.

Occasionally, a fascinating, older relative who we obediently called "Uncle" or "Aunt" would join us at the table to share exotic stories and reminisce about the good old days. Sometimes my grandfather told the tale of how, when he was just a boy my age, he left his home in Russia and journeyed alone to America.

When the stories and food were exhausted, my sister and I would belly flop onto the big overstuffed couch and fall into a restful, contented nap. The adults played cards, mostly pinochle, as hazy rings of cigar smoke floated up through the air. Later, my cousin Dennis and I wandered off in search of mischief while my older brother and cousins tossed pennies on the sidewalk and talked about girls. This ritual repeated itself week after week.

Only now do I fully grasp how Sunday's meal stirred in me a deep sense of belonging. On this day my family became whole. Of all my childhood memories, those of my family gathered around the table remain the most edifying and meaningful.

These early experiences were forgotten until the idea for a

book about the connection between food and spirituality flew suddenly into my mind like an airborne seed from a foreign land. It caught me off guard and caused surprising consequences. Like a spring river's gushing white water, it proved strong enough to wear away old ideas and carry me along on its current—a current so strong it had me, who was raised with little religious training, exploring ancient food rituals and wearing the saffron-colored robes of a Buddhist monk. Today I realize the idea's power originated in the language of my heart and awakened a part of my soul long dormant or, perhaps, just ignored.

Most actions, eating included, may be done either at a surface level or in a deeper, more thoughtful and meaningful way. Food is unique in that it offers us the tools—both personally and as a community—to transform the most ordinary morsel into the realm of the spiritual and sacred. Eating with mindfulness brings us into the moment, helps us understand what it means to be alive, and connects us to the mystery and source of all living things. Food can even unlock the door to our most personal, treasured memories.

The purpose of this book is to explore the vast number of ways that food enhances and brings meaning to life. Part I, "Spiritual Ingredients," explores how food's ancient and historic roots—as found in our wisdom traditions—help us deepen ordinary life and encounter the divine. Part II, "Our Mindful Seasonings," investigates many ancient religious and cultural rituals, prayers, and practices appropriate for both individual and family use that elevate food into the realm of the sacred. Part III, "Return to Source," surveys ancient and modern wisdom on what foods are recommended or forbidden. This includes an ecological perspective on food and eating, in addition to the "Six Steps to Changing Food Habits." Each part also offers a collection of inner meal practices, or exercises—located at the end of each chapter. These practices are designed to attune anyone, regardless of religious belief, to food's ultimate purpose: the affirmation of all life and the basis for the existence and well-being of our body, mind, and spirit.

This book, which is based upon a mindful and spiritual approach to food, offers you, as a reader, many long-term benefits. These include a newfound significance for every meal—with daily practices you can use and cultivate quietly for yourself or share with family and friends, methods for overcoming food habits and addictions, and suggestions for eating more healthfully and feeling better about your food choices. In the end, it will give you the freedom to create a new relationship with food.

So, you may be asking if this is a traditional "diet book," or whether it is a diet book at all. Strictly speaking, the answer is no. However, since the power of mindfulness increases our awareness and helps us better manage the foods we eat, let this be thought of as a book about the mindful, or spiritual diet.

Unlike other diets, this one does not attempt to control food or count calories. Instead, it affirms that as whole persons we cannot be reduced to a set of numbers. There is only being in the moment with each skillful or unskillful choice. It's really about having complete freedom to choose what is best for you at the physical, mental, and spiritual levels.

However, freedom to choose food isn't like writing a blank check. It isn't nearly as simple and easy as it appears on the surface. Instead, it derives its strength and power from a highly tuned awareness, diligent practice, and a set of practical tools that can be applied to different occasions. Rather than make food the central focus of life, the mindful diet taps into the art of using food as a personal path to greater mindfulness and spiritual connection, or metaphorically, the inner meal.

I once heard a Benedictine monk say, "If you want a quick way to see how people relate to God, watch the way they eat." I know what he said is true, because I spent the better part of my life using food as a temporary salve.

Unfortunately, it's all too easy to use food as a kind of emotional filler. This meal satisfies hunger. That meal eases loneliness. One meal promises love. Another meal lessens boredom. Today's meal soothes frustration. Tomorrow's meal offers hope. Eventually, we have to ask ourselves, "When does it ever end?" But this kind of emotional eating is food as "ordinary," as a means of quenching our basic hungers and desires. The thing is, desire wells up again as soon as the last bite is taken. Fortunately, it doesn't have to be that way.

Everything we need for a spiritual diet is available to us. Too often, however, it's hidden by a barrage of limiting, daily static about food. This static reaches us through our families, advertisements, grocery stores, restaurant menus, and so on. Fortunately, we can learn to look behind, around, and through the static. Personally, I find that setting a rhythm for the day helps me dial out the static and tune in to the clearer frequency of my own inner meal.

For example, during my stay at a cottage on monastery grounds—the place where I wrote much of this book—I follow a simple routine: I awaken while the dew remains on the grass. I wash, dress, and step outside for a twenty- to thirty-minute walking meditation. After returning to the cottage I make a small breakfast consisting of cereal, fruit, and a slice of bread with jam. Before eating, I reflect on the food in a special way—using methods that are in this book as exercises. Now I'm ready to work, feeling nourished in a way that gives me more than just the usual physical and mental strength and stamina. The food also provides a spiritual strength that feeds all aspects of my life with greater meaning.

Sometimes, for a change of pace, I venture out for a morning newspaper and a breakfast of oatmeal, fruit, and a bagel at a nearby delicatessen—I guess I still long for the spicy aroma of my grandmother's cooking. One day, a "Dear Abby" column featuring the headline "Sweet Gifts Turn Sour for Overeater" catches my attention. The letter writer describes herself as "a compulsive overeater" who has, for the first time, survived the holidays without needing to medicate her feelings with food. Her family and friends, apparently aware of her difficulties, present her with "several gifts of home-baked sweets." That's a perfect example of what I mean by "food static."

The irony is that food, when elevated to the extraordinary or sacred, provides what we need to make our lives more meaningful and complete. It strengthens family bonds, encourages love, creates a caring environment, connects us to our community, promotes a positive global outlook, sparks personal awareness, curbs negative desire, and blesses us with good health. Best of all, the opportunity to use food for increased spiritual awareness is available with every meal, every morsel, every bite.

I invite you now to come along with me—as a treasured guest—on a journey down the road to self-discovery. This journey investigates ancient methods of prayer—practices like Lectio Divina, or "divine reading"—that possess the power to transform. It defines a new kind of personal ecology—ecospirituality—from which you can fashion your spiritual development. It passes through the center of a giving heart, letting you experience the choreographed beauty of a Japanese tea ceremony. It shows how the major wisdom traditions use food as a spiritual path, including the reasons behind the recommended diets of each. It traverses many cultures and wisdom traditions, giving you the opportunity to taste from a variety of mindfulness-related rituals where hospitality, responsibility, sharing, charity, and serving coexist. It is the path of the inner meal.

As a guest on this journey, you are asked only one thing: to allow yourself to remember what has always been known, but is somehow forgotten. I like to think that each of us possesses a fully nourished, spiritual inner self. This self is centered, wise, and brimming with unlimited potential. It is not hungry, greedy, or covetous for its next meal. The challenge we face is not letting life's many distractions, problems, and details keep us from what is our awakened birthright. Once we remember this knowing place within ourselves—accomplished with centering food rituals and mindfulness—we can live in complete harmony with ourselves and others.

This remembering exists on two planes: it lives within each of us as individuals, and within our relationship to the community. Food can be used as a personal tool to liberate our consciousness or encounter God. The Buddha, for example, ate a small bowl of rice to energize his will and concentration to attain enlightenment. Food is also a communal tool—one through which we can realize compassion, love, and service for others. There is every reason for us to walk both of these roads simultaneously. To lose this sacred remembrance, however, may be to miss out on an opportunity to transform sorrow and pain into unbridled joy and wonder.

We stand today at crossroads between realities such as these. It is for us to decide how to feed the community and manifest love in the world. The *art of the inner meal* is in knowing how to make choices that are spiritually nourishing—both personally and communally.

Journeys can be strange. They seem to occur in linear fashion through time. Mine did, too, stretching over nearly two years while researching, interviewing, and learning various rituals. Yet, as sequential as that seems, I lived it in separate moments, each like a bend in the river or a colorful tile in a larger mosaic.

If the written experience feels bite-sized, know that I have written it that way intentionally. Exercises, memories, and even moments in history exist side by side, like the shifting and subtle currents in a single river. Partake of its exhilarating waters. Sit quietly by the shoreline and gaze at deep, still pools. Or close your eyes and listen to waves gently lapping at your feet. Rest the tired, weary part of your soul. After all, the journey into food's spiritual connection is one of awakening, healing, and renewal, and a remembrance of things forgotten. Luckily, I have found extraordinary help along the way.

2 – The Primal Source

We came out from the deep
To learn to love, to learn how to live
We came out from the deep
To avoid the mistakes we made.

That's why we are here!

We came out from the deep
To help and understand, but not to kill
It takes many lives till we succeed
To clear the debts of many hundreds years.

That's why we are here!

—Enigma, lyrics from "Out From The Deep"

Long shadows of a eucalyptus tree are cast over damp, uneven grass. The night's condensation drips water from a white-painted porch overhang onto the pavement. I step slowly, feeling the coolness of the ground beneath my feet. Through barren branches the sun alternately sparkles and disappears from my vision with each step of my walking meditation. Evidence of the living, breathing

Earth is all around, and it is hard to believe that there are times when we do not, or cannot, notice.

Food, too, offers conclusive evidence of our interconnectedness to living nature. It gives us life, breath, and consciousness. In our midst, like an ancient broth prepared by wise shamans and prophets, there exist timeless stories of this connection. To deepen our awareness of this primal source of nourishment, we need only to sip from the spiritual broth of Pagan, or primal religions, and wisdom traditions that use food to inform us of our sacred place in the cosmos.

An ancient parable from Hindu scriptures uses the staple of salt to explain how the divine lives within each of us. The story goes like this: a wise father asks his son, who is conceited and puffed up with his knowledge of scripture, to place salt into a bowl of water. The father then asks the son to find the now dissolved salt. When the young man cannot find it, his father tells him to taste water from the middle and ends of the bowl. The son soon discovers that the salt resides everywhere, though it can't easily be perceived. He learns the lesson that salt, like the divine spirit, though not easily perceived, resides in all things.

We, too, can use the "salt" that is all around us to season our daily meal. In doing so we discover not only the eternal spirit within the Earth, but within ourselves. The primal religions—even the Paganism practiced today—teach us very much this same basic lesson: that through nature we can directly experience the living will and expression of divinity. This lesson is relevant because it lets us honor and respect the Earth—and also appreciate an important part of our past.

For much of human history, nature was not viewed as something distinct and separate from God. Nature was a direct manifestation of the divine, one that often took the female form. Before the advent of machines and technology, when human survival depended on a budding and fragile agriculture for survival, the deities of fertility were frequently called upon to ensure a successful harvest. As such, Mother Creator, Mother Corn, Earth Goddess, and others were givers of life and sources of unbounded creativity and love. The myths surrounding such figures have remained constant over the centuries.

Long before we witnessed Earth from the emptiness of outer space, the concept of Earth as a wholly integrated, living spiritual essence was ingrained in the human psyche. The ancient Greeks regaled in this spirit thousands of years ago:

> *Gaia*
> *mother of all,*
> *foundation of all,*
> *the oldest one.*
>
> *I shall sing to Earth.*
> *She feeds everything*
> *that is in the world...*
>
> *Queen of Earth*
> *through you*
> *beautiful children,*
> *beautiful harvests come.*
>
> *The giving of life*
> *and the taking of life,*
>
> *both are yours.*
>
> —"Hymn to Gaia" (as translated in *The Essential Mystics* by Andrew Harvey)

Such primal beliefs still resonate today. Some Native American traditions, for example, include the practice of passing over the first of any plant and harvesting the second. What a beautiful practice in an era of the machine, where living food products are reduced to units. Like those before us, we can practice walking gently on the land. We can strive to take only what we need and leave something behind for others. Born of Mother Goddess, should we not respect, love, and care for her as she cares for us?

There are many ways that the spirit of the Earth speaks to us. We all experience awe-inspiring sights and sounds of Earth that take our breath away. These are felt on a grand scale, as when we witness the massive depth, scope, and colors of the Grand Canyon. They are also felt on a small scale, in each morsel of food on our plate. Is the miracle of food any less amazing? Does not each grape, apple, and orange speak to us of our dependence on the Earth? When you pick up your food at the market, as most of us do, it's easy to forget that humankind has been grounded or connected to the soil for most of our history. The *art of the inner meal* begins here—with respect, reverence, and appreciation for the soil that brings us life.

Many primal religions—both past and present—have utilized this concept of sacred ground as a mainstay of their world view. Centuries ago, for example, pre-Islamic Arabs gathered around sacred standing stones—found at Mecca and other sites—through which they communed with God, Goddess, and other deities. Today, there are African tribes that place standing stones outside their living quarters for protection and good luck. In some Native American traditions, creation is the result of a primal substance—called *inyan*—that shapes reality and manifests itself through rock and stone. One tribe, the Oneida, are even known as "the people of the Oneida stone."

At a deep level, we still feel comforted by the mysterious and primal power of Earth.

What Is Your Inner Meal Path?

It is afternoon. The winter sun spreads an unusually warm blanket of light in through the cottage windows. I pause from my writing to watch two saffron-robed monks remove an old tree stump. City bred for most of my life, I am surprised at how incredibly well anchored it is. The stump is only about one foot in diameter, but the hole the monks dig reveals four impressive major roots jutting out from the stump's core. Acting as stabilizers, each of these roots looks as large, if not larger, than the stump itself. I cannot help but wonder: How many of Earth's marvels are buried beneath the earth or the sea, or occur out of our sight? How many are invisibly anchored and grounded in depths beyond our comprehension?

Humankind's wisdom traditions are not unlike the leafy maple trees that populated the midwestern forests I frequented as a youth. We experience and witness our traditions, like the branches of a tree, through what we can see, feel, touch, taste, and hear: rituals, churches, temples, symbols, chants, prayers, foods, meditations, and so on. In reality, these are all deeply rooted and nourished by myth, history, lore, legend, wisdom, faith, and knowledge—even, perhaps, unconscious memory—that go back several millennia. The ancient Jewish religion, for example, was notably influenced by the ideas of the Greeks and others, especially in the area of food. Paul William Roberts, author of *In Search of the Birth of Jesus* writes: "The purity and dietary laws of the Jews as well as other ritual meals, the prayers with their tying of cords, and the celebrating of feasts, can all be traced to the profound influence exerted by Zoroastrianism on Judaism during the Babylonian exile." In some sense, we are still connected to the ancient, primal source.

Whatever your religious affiliation, background, or tradition, you have a unique opportunity to create a personalized inner meal path. You need only draw upon the diverse sources of wisdom and knowledge that strengthen the bond between food, mindfulness, and spirituality.

For Hindus, food provides a means through which one may discover the true self. For Buddhists, it offers a path toward liberated consciousness, moderation, and loving-kindness. For Jews, food brings the innate holiness and wholesomeness of each moment to life. For Christians, it brings the essence of communion into the community through service and love. For Muslims, it provides a means for surrendering to God's will.

Choose from among any or all of these traditions to attain your faith's highest core ideals and aspirations. For, as the philosopher Huston Smith writes, "It is possible to climb life's mountain from any side, but when the top is reached the trails converge...Is life not more interesting for the varied contributions of Confucianists, Taoists, Buddhists, Muslims, Jews, and Christians?"

The inner meal path is not so different from any spiritual path with heart. I recall, for example, the story about a man whose path was the act of greeting people. Whenever there was a knock on the door he would say, "The Lord is at the door." He reached his faith's ideals by seeing God in everybody. The inner meal is like that; it lets us see the work of the divine in each morsel of food.

In broader terms, embarking on the inner meal path teaches us tolerance and respect for the differences that exist between traditions. In reality, they are not so different after all. At their heart beats a common purpose, like that stated so simply and eloquently in the Bible's Book of Micah:

> *And what does the Lord require of you*
> *but to do justice, and to love kindness,*
> *and to walk humbly with your God?*

PRACTICE: REFLECTION ON MOTHER EARTH

The purpose of this exercise is to delve into the mysteries that unfold when we ask ourselves, "What is the nature of this planet we walk upon each day? What is Mother Earth?"

Use this exercise whenever you have a free moment to bask in the wonder of nature's myriad connections—each a complex strand in the web of life. May you enjoy many such moments.

Take some time to find a rock, tree, or plant that feels special. Maybe it's the hibiscus on the patio that brightens your day each time it flowers, or the orange tree that you've picked sweet fruit from, or the stone that you've noticed from time to time. Sit or stand nearby and simply watch it for a few minutes as you reflect. How long has it been there? How does it contribute to the surroundings? How does its presence enable the lives of insects, birds, and other living things?

Try to sense into the cycle of life that these objects and nature are part of. To feel this is to know the connection between ourselves and all of life.

The benefits of this reflection on nature are many. It helps us become conscious of the link between the food that we eat and the Earth from which it grows. It gives us respect for nature—with all its grandeur, complexity, and subtleness. It helps us appreciate the blessings and bounty that Earth provides for us all. By awakening our connection to the soil, we can better understand our responsibility as primary guardian of the nourishing Earth. Finally, it lets us gain a deeper understanding of the primal source from which all our treasured wisdom traditions are nourished.

PRACTICE: FOOD INVENTORY

A food inventory is a useful way to connect to early memories of food and eating. It is also a valuable tool for exploring how your food likes and dislikes have changed over the years. This practice may help you become more aware of how your eating has evolved.

To complete this exercise, take a sheet of paper and divide it into five columns. In the first column, write down the foods you remember eating during childhood (ages 1-10). Beside each food item, you can add a plus (+) or minus (-) sign to denote whether you liked or disliked that particular food.

In the second column, list those foods that were part of your diet during your adolescent and teenage years (11-19).

In the third column, write down the foods you ate during your young adult years (20-29).

The fourth column will include those items you eat presently as an adult. In addition to foods that make up the basis of your daily food intake, don't forget to include items that you crave for and eat on a periodic basis.

The final column represents your ideal diet. Here, write down those foods that you think would benefit your physical, emotional, and spiritual health and well-being. This column may include foods you currently eat. Or it may include foods you rarely, if ever, eat. This is your chance to be more discriminating, without worrying about your desires.

After you finish filling in all the columns, look at the trends and patterns. Do you notice anything? Most likely, your eating choices have changed and evolved over time. If not, then you might want to ask yourself why this is so? At what time period in your life did your food choices become locked or frozen?

It is not unusual for our present choices to be linked to the past. I remember one woman, Janice (not her real name) who listed peanuts in every food column because that was her father's favorite food. While some of us cherish mementos handed down by our parents, others use food as a keepsake. Another woman, Mary, listed condensed milk in the "adult" column. She had recently discovered it, and she loved the feeling of comfort it gave her. But when Mary mentioned this to her mother, she got a big surprise. Her mother commented that when Mary was a baby, she was often fed condensed milk!

The benefits of this exercise are many. It may lead to new connections between your present and past food choices. A food inventory may also reveal emotional connections to food. Perhaps most importantly, it may give you concrete evidence that you have changed your food habits before, and that you can do it again. Remember, eating mindfully doesn't mean you can't enjoy food. But it might mean that you can savor each bite more completely—so you can fulfill yourself in moderation, rather than fill yourself up.

3 – Finding True Self

Oh, the wonder of joy!
I am the food of life,
and I am he who eats the food of life:
I am the two in ONE.
I am the first-born of the world of truth,
born before the gods,
born in the center of immortality.
He who gives me is my salvation.
I am that food which eats the eater of food.

—Translated by Juan Mascaró,
Taittiriya Upanishad, 3.10.6

From Food Desire to True Self

For the Hindu, food constitutes an essential part of our training here on Earth. It is even assumed that at some point we will enjoy the pleasures of the flesh and certainly overindulge in food! The world we inhabit is one of *maya,* or illusion—purposely filled with tasty delicacies and other illusory pleasures to set in motion our basic and most advanced spiritual lessons. As human beings, we live in a state of duality, set in motion by and bound to our ego's earthly desires, which separate us from our true Self or God.

Hinduism believes that this knowledge of true Self and the human liberation from a cycle of birth and death is attainable, and what's more, personal transcendence is the one true goal of life. The inner meal path offers us a means for approaching this highest ideal.

Hinduism's roots trace back over four thousand years to the Vedas and even more ancient oral traditions. One part of Hindu scripture, the Upanishads, refers to the Tree of Eternity that extends from heaven down to the Earth. Within this eternity, the Earth derives its physical nature from the three basic *gunas*, or primal energies that form the universe.

The three *gunas*—known in Sanskrit as *sattva*, *rajas*, and *tamas*—bring certain qualities and forces to bear on all of nature, including humans and food. Since food, for example, comprises the condensed vibratory energy of these *gunas*, we absorb each food's innate energy properties whenever we eat.

Do you become drowsy, edgy, or alert after eating? The energy properties of food—discussed in chapter 13—may be accountable. According to the Hindu perspective, tamasic-based foods make us slow, dull, lazy, and weak; rajasic-based foods propel us toward action, ambition, and hunger; sattvic-based foods create in us balance, purity, and composure. Paramahansa Yogananda, in his commentary *God Talks with Arjuna: The Bhagavad Gita*, writes: "Modern scientists analyze the value of foodstuffs according to their physical properties and how they react on the body; but yogis, who anciently delved in the spiritual science of food, consider its vibratory nature in determining what is beneficial, stimulating, or harmful when ingested."

The *gunas* can be thought of as more than energy. In ancient lore they are what cause our actions and thoughts take root:

> *There is a fig tree*
> *In ancient story,*
> *The giant Aswattha,*
> *The everlasting,*
> *Rooted in heaven,*

Its branches earthward:
Each of its leaves
Is a song of the Vedas,
And he who knows it
Knows all the Vedas.

Downward and upward
Its branches bending
Are fed by the gunas,
The buds it puts forth
Are the things of the senses,
Roots it has also
Reaching downward
Into this world,
The roots of man's action.

—the *Bhagavad-Gita* (translated by Prabhavananda and Isherwood)

It is, therefore, our very human, insatiable desire that plunges us into food's special pleasures of taste and smell. Only after desire causes enough pain, leaves us empty, and fails to satisfy us deeply do we try a more fruitful path—one in which food is used for its special properties that can either hinder or help our spiritual development. Hinduism recognizes that the path to self-discovery and God varies according to each person's unique temperament and nature. Four kinds of yoga are available to achieve the goal of union with God. Whatever method or practice of yoga one uses, the emphasis is always on building up one's spiritual strength slowly through increased awareness. This practice of slowly building up strength relates to food as well.

For example, I always had a weakness for sweets. In the past, I didn't have sufficient awareness or strength to stop eating when I wanted. If I so much as took one little bite of a chocolate chip cookie, custard pastry, scoop of cherry vanilla ice cream, or a piece of peanut brittle, then there was no stopping me until I ate all that remained. It seemed that the more I resisted, the more I was unable to resist. I was no closer to changing my eating habits than a zebra was to turning in his stripes.

Sometimes, I'd even make an impulsive trip to the store for more until my immediate hunger was satisfied. As bad as the lump in my stomach made me feel afterward, the lump of regret and guilt was even worse. The guilt stayed with me far longer than my unhealthy habits. Rather than helping me avoid another binge of sweets, it might have caused me to repeat the behavior. That's because guilt does not activate awareness; it only serves to feed anxiety and fuel more compulsive behavior. What I didn't know at the time was that one way to slowly build up strength and resistance—to food or to anything—is through heightened awareness.

Awareness or Ignorance?

The Hindu concept of *karma*, the universe's direct law of moral cause and effect, is intriguing in relation to food. According to the law of karma, every action begets an equal reaction. It's not just what we eat that matters, but *how*. Food treated as "ordinary," eaten with greed and hunger, produces a karmic reaction with consequences that its misuse can burden us with in this lifetime, if not the next reincarnation. The right food, eaten while reflecting on its benefits to our temple of consciousness—the body—produce no adverse karmic reaction. These decisions are ours alone to make, once we possess total freedom of choice. Yet, how can we exercise freedom of choice if we are not truly aware?

Whether or not you believe in reincarnation, the struggle we face daily to choose between the foods that are good for us and those that are bad, but often delectable, is a real one. During workshops, I often use the phrase "your karma is in the refrigerator." Most people get it right away. After all, haven't we all experienced how our food choices produce a measurable cause and effect on our bodies? The food we eat changes the way we look and the way we feel. It can even change our moods. Just ask your doctor; he or she will tell you that improper diet can result in high cholesterol, diabetes, gout, heart disease, ulcers, and a host of other problems.

Here's a quick way to gauge your present state of mindful eating. When your doctor tells you that you need to change your eating habits, what do you do? Do you actively seek out a better diet? Or do you procrastinate and conveniently forget the advice, hoping the problem will go away? I know a man who, instead of finding a more evolved way of eating, finds another doctor instead. The problem with nonawareness is that it never makes bad news get better or disappear for very long.

The same never-ending struggle between awareness and ignorance is a theme throughout Indian and Hindu literature. One of that tradition's most revered writings is the more than 2,220-year-old Bhagavad Gita, or the Song of God. The Bhagavad Gita centers on a battle about to be waged by Prince Arjuna. Arjuna is disconsolate at having to fight, but does so only at the urging of the divine Krishna.

That the divine Lord Krishna encourages his spiritual disciple to engage in battle seems incredible until we realize, as Prabhavananda points out in *The Spiritual Heritage of India,* "that the way of realizing divine consciousness, and attaining eternal life and infinite peace, is through complete detachment and self-surrender. We can understand the Gita as a holy scripture and Krishna as a divine teacher only when we consider that this war is but an occasion for bringing spiritual truths to our attention."

Arjuna's battle, like that which we sometimes have with food, can be interpreted as a metaphorical one. It's really representative of the ongoing struggle within ourselves, and nothing more. We can remain unaware and refuse to fight our inner demons, or we can take up the fight and awaken to the indulgences and habits that bind us in place. Spiritual achievement is gained through practice, and sometimes it feels as if we're fighting a war—although the "enemy" is ourselves.

Paramahansa Yogananda draws a distinction between the body and mind that dwell together. He tells us that by treating our body with the utmost care and respect, we also honor and respect our inner Spirit:

Mutilation or any excessive 'punishment' of the physical form is condemned by the Bhagavad Gita. Man's true enemy is not his body but his mind. His so-called physical passions are in reality produced by dark mental forces—anger, greed, lust, which all men on the spiritual path must try to subdue and conquer.

The body is the materialization of the indwelling life and consciousness of Spirit as the individualized soul. The nature of Spirit is purity and harmony; beauty, vitality, and radiance. To abuse the body in any way that distorts this image is to offend the Creator Lord by disfiguring his human masterpiece.

Breaking Free from Habits and Desire

Have you ever tried changing an eating behavior or even an addiction? If so, then you're like most of us who know how difficult it is to alter even small or annoying surface habits, like taking that extra slice of cake or oversnacking. It's enough to make one wonder: Is the habit in control of me, or am I in control of the habit?

Eating habits don't change overnight. Knowledge and understanding of food's ultimate purpose take time. Breaking the chains of desire can take even longer, making it quite easy to return to earlier patterns of behavior. Familiar territory always feels comfortable until you find greater comfort elsewhere. So, where do we begin? How do we break unwanted habits?

I once asked a friend of mine, a monk, if he thought it was possible to change deeply embedded habits or addictions. He answered cryptically, "It is both possible, and impossible."

The "possible" allows us to change our actions—either the action of eating or any other habit—by engaging our determination and will. This is illustrated in an Asian proverb that says that although you can judge the value of a diamond by looking at its physical qualities, you can't judge a person simply by looking at their physical appearance. To really know someone you need to grasp the depth and quality of their will, heart, and mind. Yet determination and willpower, while important, may not be enough to change habits, and even hypnotists suggest that willpower can be easily overcome. That's where the "impossible" comes into play.

Changing long-embedded habits is impossible *unless* we first activate our awareness. We may still react compulsively, but dawning awareness undermines and weakens the foundation of compulsion. Through awareness we begin to gain strength of will and self-observation. It helps us approach life from that place within us where strength resides, not weakness.

Awareness lets us feel a habit's presence, its hold on us, and maybe the reasons for its arising. Once fully aware, we can short-circuit habits by engaging our determination, understanding what benefits the change provides for us, and lastly, by substituting a satisfying new action to replace the old. No habit changes unless we deeply understand that food is the essential nutrient for our mind, body, and spirit.

To read Jack Kerouac's *On The Road* is to almost believe that his diet was the unintentional inspiration for his frenetic, hopped-up writing style. Shortly after Kerouac leaves New York for the West Coast, we learn about his favorite food habit. In Illinois: "Along about three in the afternoon, after an apple pie and ice cream in a roadside stand, a woman stopped for me in a little coupe." In Davenport, Iowa: "I ate another apple pie and ice cream; that's practically all I ate all the way across the country, I knew it was nutritious and it was delicious, of course." In Des Moines: "I ate apple pie and ice cream—it was getting better as I got deeper into Iowa, the pie bigger, the ice cream richer." But being conscious of *what* you like—as Kerouac was—is not the same as knowing *why* you like something.

Awareness puts a magnifying glass to our actions and the thoughts that give voice to our desires. This is self-observation at a deep level, and it is activated when we consciously set an intention to observe ourselves—without blame or judgment. This intention can be set anytime, anywhere—before or during a meal, for example.

This process takes time, however, so don't be surprised if initially you don't notice a habit or a thought until after it begins, or even after it finishes. Actions of the mind and body can be *extremely* subtle. If you find that self-observation stops, just note this to yourself, and once again state your intention to observe your actions and thoughts. As you practice observing your mind, you'll begin to detect the kind of impulsive and habit-forming ideas and desires that whet your appetite in the first place.

In observing habits, guilt is not an issue. Letting guilt into your life is like letting a ghost from the past control your actions in the present. This does not mean you don't recognize that a particular habit may be harmful to yourself or others; after all, that is why you are trying to change it. Allow yourself, as in the Hindu tradition, to enjoy food habits while also realizing their bothersome aspects. Again, be easy on yourself; you are acting only as a detective, and no crime has been committed! So the next time you feel guilty, just observe the guilt. As you become more aware, you'll experience the joy and bliss inherent in every meal.

Hindu sage Vivekananda, in *The Practical Vedanta*, tells us that our perception of weakness is self-generated. We need only remove our hands from our eyes to let in the light and see the true self within—a self that is fully aware:

> *Millions of years have passed since man first came here, and yet but one infinitesimal part of his powers has been manifested. Therefore, you must not say that you are weak. How do you know what possibilities lie behind that degradation on the surface? You know little of that which is within you. For behind you is the ocean of infinite power and blessedness.*

A Spiritual Meal Guideline

Spiritual meals, whatever their tradition, contain much in common. Almost all, for example, utilize ritual cleansing and prayer. But

while these meals—described at the end of chapters 3 through 7—
basically follow the same pattern, you will find substantial differences in emphasis and meaning.

A spiritual meal in the Hindu and Indian tradition taps into
the spirit of enjoying food by giving hospitality to others. In India, the sharing of food—at a festival, at home, or at a wedding—
is woven into the fabric of how people express their joy and
happiness at appropriate and opportune occasions. To experience the essence of such a spiritual meal, try to incorporate the
following steps.

Respect Your Guests. Showing respect to guests is an essential part of Hindu and Indian tradition. The Hindu belief that
God resides within each person means that each guest should be
honored, welcomed, and entertained with special care. For either a
meal or a short visit, hospitality usually begins by offering guests a
cup of sweet, milky black or spiced tea.

Begin With a Prayer. Reciting a prayer over the meal does
more than bring family and friends together. For example, a blessing
by Swami Paramanda—from his *Book of Daily Thoughts and Prayer*—
connects us to the ultimate purpose of food with these words:

> *May the Lord accept this, our offering, and bless our food
> that it may bring us strength in our body, vigor in our
> mind, and selfless devotion in our heart for his service.*

A mealtime prayer also benefits us by calming us down so we
can enjoy our meal and more fully digest our food.

Enjoy Your Meal. Some Hindu sects eat vegetarian meals,
mainly to avoid harming animals. Historically, meat-eating and honoring guests by the slaughtering of a cow was practiced among
certain Brahmin castes. Ironically, it was this cruel treatment
of animals and other abuses that, in the sixth century B.C.,
led two Brahmin-born princes—the Buddha and Mahavira, the
founder of Jainism—to embrace a more compassionate and
nonviolent diet.

Whether or not your meal is vegetarian, be aware of the wonderful bounty of food before you. Enjoy your scrumptious meal's many tastes, aromas, and flavors. Offer it graciously and as a gift of love to others.

Eat With Awareness. While enjoying your food, you can still be fully aware of your desires. By observing your desires you'll eventually gain the strength to resist foods that are not in your best interests.

Make a point of eating an occasional meal in silence. This will help you feel the profound connection between the food you eat—sattvic, rajasic, or tamasic-based—and its effect on your life energy, mindfulness, and physical health. From this inner meal practice of awareness you plant the seed of finding the true self.

PRACTICE: AWARENESS AND OBSERVING

There are many methods for finding your way back to the inner meal path should you ever lose your way. Simple awareness, or "observing," is a good way to embrace the path, remain on solid ground, and grow beyond unhealthy eating habits. It's a fundamental practice that keeps you in touch with your path.

By cultivating awareness, you're not trying to change any habits. You're not even judging yourself. You simply observe or witness the desire or action with a sense of detachment—as if you are watching it on TV or hearing someone else tell you about it. Come back and use this practice anytime that you feel you're not properly managing your eating.

One way to begin to open your awareness channels is to close your eyes and repeat these words: *May my all-knowing self allow me to observe my behavior so that I may attain freedom of choice.* Or you might try writing down the action

---

you want to observe. This alerts your unconscious mind to be on the lookout for the offending habit. If repeating these words feels forced, just allow yourself to nonverbally know of your intent to be aware.

For the actual observation, simply state your habit matter-of-factly in your mind as it appears. If Kerouac had witnessed his eating habits while on the road, he might have thought, "Eating vanilla ice cream. Eating hot apple pie. Tasting the ice cream and the apple and crust of the pie." You can even describe the feeling of hunger or desire you feel during the action—for example, "I feel my hunger for ice cream. I desire its sweet creamy taste. I like the coolness and smoothness in my mouth. I taste it and I want more."

You can also observe and become aware of your surroundings. Is there something about a place, a feeling, or a situation that connects you to food? What do you feel as you sit down to a meal? Maybe you're eating because you're tired, nervous, frustrated, bored, hurt, angry, anxious, happy, fearful, or sad.

Allow yourself to observe the emotion that precedes or accompanies the habit. Don't even try to change the particular emotion. Simply recognize and become familiar with it. Connect with it, but do so with a sense of detachment and separation. You might find yourself saying matter-of-factly, "I'm eating to calm myself down. I'm nervous. I need to feel comforted and relaxed."

Building up mindfulness means letting yourself feel your desires, not repressing them. Eventually, you will have the strength to resist or say no even though you desire a particular food.

After each meal or experience, tape-record or write down your account of having witnessed the behavior. When you have finished recording your witnessing, permit yourself, like Prince Arjuna in the Bhagavad Gita, to awaken to the true Self that loves and accepts you with total compassion.

A deep awareness offers many positive side benefits. It brings us into the present moment where we really live our lives. It allows us to open ourselves up to change. It helps us develop tolerance and a nonjudgmental attitude. It lets us realize that we and our habits are not the same. It builds up our strength and resistance to unhealthy foods. It gives us the freedom of choice we need to alter our diet in a positive and life-affirming way.

4 – Liberation, Moderation, and Loving-Kindness

awoke this morning
to find that my people's tongues were tied
and in my dreams
they were given books to poison their minds.
the river is deep and the mountain high,
how long before the other side.

we are their mortar,
their building bricks and their clay.
their gold teeth mirror
both our joys and our pain.
the river is deep and the ocean wide,
who will teach us how to read the signs.

—Dead Can Dance, lyrics from "Song of the Dispossessed"

During my morning walking meditation beside a large meadow, thousands of dew-tipped blades of grass sparkle like crystal white diamonds. These are but a few of the jewels spread all around us each moment of the day. Sometimes, discovering these jewels is just a matter of reflecting on our surroundings with a fresh set of eyes.

Because we eat many meals each day, and many thousands of meals in a lifetime, it's easy to forget the specialness of the moment. Eating is never mundane, however, as long as the plate of food before us serves as a jewel of awakened consciousness and compassion. This was definitely the case for a man who came out of northeast India over twenty-five hundred years ago bearing a unique message.

Born a Prince, Siddhartha Gautama renounced his privileged background and went into the forest to seek enlightenment. Several years later while meditating under the Bodhi tree—the tree of enlightenment—he attained his goal. This was the beginning of forty-five years of traveling the countryside as the Buddha, or "The Awakened One" as he was now called, to spread the word of liberated consciousness, or ultimate reality. The Buddha's message did not rely on the Hindu Vedic scriptures. Instead, he stressed that by leading the right kind of life one could light the lamp of awakening in one's own soul. "Be a lamp unto yourselves," was the Buddha's constant refrain.

A fascinating creation story is described within the voluminous tens of thousands of pages of the Buddha's discourses, or *suttas*—the Pali word for the Sanskrit *sutras*. In that story, food plays a major part. According to the *Aggañña Sutta*, or *Discourse on Genesis*, life on Earth developed from a process of evolution taking millions of years. The world evolved into a beautiful garden of living things, populated with divine beings who were half human and half angel. These first humans possessed *jana*, a superconsciousness of radiance, purity, and calmness. With their janic power, they flew effortlessly through space, experienced heavenly bliss, and needed no physical food to survive. This blissful state continued until the day one of the angels, out of curiosity, tasted Earth's most tempting food—a very delicious, sweet, creamy white nectar, *rasa pathavi*, which in the Buddha's native language of Pali means "taste of the Earth."

It was in this moment that the unwholesome mental states of attachment, greed, and desire first arose. As angels hoarded and fought over this sweet taste of the Earth they gained more physical desires. Eventually, the fallen angels lost their divine bliss to become the humans we are today—people grounded in suffering rooted in desire and the impermanence of all things.

The Buddha taught that by leading a wholesome life human beings can attain spiritual power and recover their previously lost divine nature. It is in this sense that the inner meal path leads to Buddhism's highest ideals. While food is the original source of desire, greed, and anger, it also is a source of nourishment by which the soul progresses. Through food humans learn the wholesome mental states of mindfulness, nonattachment, loving-kindness, self-control, compassion, and appreciation of Earth as the common heritage of all people and all living things.

In Buddhism, food can be eaten to satisfy hunger and desire, or to liberate conscious awareness. The latter makes food sacred because we make a connection regarding the interdependency between food and long life, and between food and awakened consciousness. By practicing the Noble Eightfold Path—Right Understanding, Right Thought, Right Speech, Right Action, Right Livelihood, Right Effort, Right Mindfulness, and Right Concentration—humans can transcend suffering and attain *nibbana*, or liberation from desire, greed, and the cycle of birth and death.

Food's "Middle Way"

Food taught the Buddha one of his most critical lessons—the importance of the "Middle Way," or moderation. It is a lesson about the inner meal path as well. Prior to the Buddha's enlightenment, he practiced a type of severe renunciation used by the ascetics of his day. This meant reducing food intake to a minimum and fasting almost continuously. After years of futility and near starvation he realized that without food there could be no physical, mental, or spiritual growth. Only after he abandoned this extreme and ate a meal of rice for nourishment did he gain enough strength to concentrate and reach enlightenment. The Buddha interpreted this to mean that there is a Middle Way between the extremes of excess and abstinence.

I'm sure you have heard or known of someone who practices extreme eating habits. The problem with extremes is that they tend to rule our lives. Almost anything can be taken to an extreme: diets, vegetarianism, meatism, healthism, and gourmandism. This raises some interesting questions: How attached are you to your "ism" and its resulting actions? Does a particular "ism" really serve your mind, body, and spirit?

> *Those whose compulsions are gone, who are not attached to food, whose sphere is emptiness, signlessness, and liberation, are hard to track, like birds in the sky.*

—Buddha, the *Dhammapada*

By "hard to track" the Buddha means free to follow our own path. A mind that is not "tracked" is not predestined, like a train, to rigidly follow tracks laid down at some previous point in time. To be "hard to track" means journeying into the present moment, without an idea of our exact termination point. If you have ever had to solve problems "on the fly" then you've experienced this kind of "hard to track" aliveness. At times like these some of our most inspired and creative solutions can take place. This is the case, too, when we allow ourselves to experience the freedom that exists between extremes, be they excess or abstinence.

There is a big difference between actions that represent self-control, commitment, and discipline, and those that are extreme. The dictionary's definition of addiction is: "To surrender oneself habitually or compulsively to something," which is to be attached to it beyond will or reason. Attachment keeps a habit or addiction firmly rooted. By using the inner meal practices of moderation and nonattachment we gently learn to let go of extremes. Compulsions and extremes lack heart and compassion, but witnessing our actions without judgment encourages both nonattachment and compassion—for ourselves and others.

As a seventeen-year-old freshman at Northwestern University in Evanston, Illinois, I started lifting weights as a hobby. I didn't know it at the time, but it was really a way to escape from the pressures and expectations put upon me to achieve high grades. As it turned out, my grades didn't improve, but my weight lifting did! I progressed quickly, and before the year was over I bench pressed more weight than most of the football players in my dormitory. My workout schedule soon became a priority that was rigidly set. I learned from more advanced weight lifters what routines I should follow—and what foods I should eat to gain maximum strength.

One weight lifter in particular had set national records in power lifting. I remember feeling as though I was finally a member of the "club" on the day he asked me to "spot" him, or stand over him in case he needed assistance, during a four-hundred-plus pound bench press. Yet this club's focus was so narrow that very little mattered other than building more muscle. Many of the best weight lifters of that time downed handfuls of supplementary vitamins and protein-laden drinks. Some routinely used a steady diet of dangerous steroids. I never flirted with steroids, but I gulped my share of protein shakes and extra vitamins.

Anyone who becomes a slave to a particular idea—whether it's building muscle or climbing Mount Everest—also risks being blind to the costs. I wonder what long-term damage many of us risk when we sacrifice the middle road to reach an extreme end. I'm not saying you shouldn't have outrageous, wild, and wonderful goals. By all means, do. The point is that by using the middle road you can reach your goals safely and with less potential harm. Herein lies the beauty of the art of the inner meal.

The Buddha's teachings—as written in the *Ovada Patimakkha*, or *Advice of the Buddha*—appear deceptively simple and straightforward, but in the real world they are not that easy:

To cultivate the good... To purify one's mind... Patience... Right speech, harmlessness, restraint... Moderation in food... Dwelling in peaceful and quiet places... [and] Striving for spiritual advancements is the teaching of all Buddhas.

Taming the Mind

Simply attempting to eat in moderation requires taming the mind, with all its wildness and desires. This is the equivalent of taming a tiger, a fiercely independent animal with a large hunger and a short attention span. Once liberated from attachment to habit and temptation, you are free to eat with awareness. You will begin to see foods with a fresh set of eyes, and be awake to which foods are nutritious, healthful, energizing, and beneficial to your entire being.

I can still recall, for example, the struggle I faced during my first twenty-four hours as a Buddhist monk—for that was when my monk's vows and the ability of food to increase spiritual strength were put to the test. As my initiation ceremony takes place on monastery grounds, I fear that a lifetime of unconscious eating and heavily ingrained habits gleefully wait in ambush.

Moving past three small banana palms, I and two other monk initiates pace slowly toward a large square of Persian rugs located on a flat, grassy field. The setting sun casts a soft orange glow over us as we repeat ancient Pali chants, answer questions, and take our monk's vows—including a vow not to eat any food past noon. Finally, the sun fades and long fingers of shadow envelop us. It is done.

My sole possessions now consist of my robes and a large lacquered bowl with a glossy black sheen. My freshly shaved head bowed, I slowly walk past a small group of devotees who provide offerings: a pair of burgundy-colored socks, a washcloth, a bar of soap, a vial of shampoo. I can't imagine what I'm going to do with the shampoo.

A monk ushers me to a small room intended for novice monks.

The eldest among us gets the bed. We younger novices choose between two small futons on the floor, each adorned with bright, red rose-patterned sheets—the only cheerful image in the room. A lone fluorescent lamp, dangling amid pale white peeling paint, glares down upon us. Thin, yellowed shades cover the windows.

I contemplate my vows when suddenly the gravity of what I have done dawns upon me. Here I am sitting cross-legged, swathed in uneven mounds and folds of orange fabric. Have I forsaken my heritage? Not only am I out of my element, but I am overwhelmed by what I don't know about Buddhism and about being a monk. Suddenly, all of my fears and doubts coalesce and converge, focusing my awareness onto what feels like the sharp tip of a needle. That needle tip pierces my consciousness and produces awareness of a temptation, sitting regally atop a shelf: there, fully intact, rests a giant-sized Cadbury's milk chocolate bar. It's about a foot from my futon. And my nose. I swear that it's smiling at me.

For a brief moment, I glance over to my monk roommates. One lies down, eyes closed. The other sits in a perfect lotus position, legs crossed, methodically clicking prayer beads between his fingers. I wonder if any of the monks would notice it missing. After all, I muse, it's only *chocolate.* Then I remember one of my recent vows—*do not take that which is not given.*

This room, I think, is big enough for the two of us—my desires and my awareness—with neither having to blot out the other. I fluff the pillows behind my back, sit up, close my eyes, and breathe deeply. For the moment, I claim a small victory. I know that tomorrow, however, brings more desire and temptation...

The Step of Loving-Kindness

You may want to further your inner meal path through practicing the Buddha's unconditional loving-kindness. Along with compassion, loving-kindness manifests through an enlightened way of being and an approach to life that embraces and transmits goodwill toward all living beings. One powerful way to experience it is through taking action. You can do this, for example, by taking on the responsibility of feeding others. This might mean getting involved in food projects to relieve hunger and suffering in your own neighborhood.

Zen Buddhist Master Bernard Glassman, coauthor of *Instructions to the Cook: A Zen Master's Lessons in Living a Life That Matters*, dedicates his life to an engaged Buddhism that includes establishing bakeries and other projects to feed and house the poor. "In Zen," says Glassman, "a vow is not something we promise to do and then feel bad or guilty about if we don't accomplish it. Rather, a vow is an *intention* to do something...By itself, a vow is all potential. It's like yeast or starter. But if we want to manifest in the world, if we want to bake a real loaf of bread, one that we can eat ourselves and serve to others, we have to add flour and water and knead them all together. We have to add determination."

A Spiritual Meal Guideline

Experiencing a spiritual meal in the Buddhist tradition means living and eating in a way that manifests compassion and loving-kindness. By following the suggestions here, you'll bring awareness, liberated consciousness, and wholesomeness to each meal and morsel.

While some Buddhist traditions require exclusively vegetarian meals, others permit meat. The Buddha himself ate meat when it was offered to him. Yet, in what was probably both a practical and compassionate decision, he taught that while it is a sin to kill for meat, it is not a sin to eat it.

Wash the Hands. It is customary in Buddhism to cleanse the hands before eating.

Begin with a Prayer. The *Vinaya Pitaka*, or *Book of Discipline*, offers a reflection on food. While it's often recited by monks, anyone can gain value by reciting it before mealtime:

With appreciation I am going to eat; not to frolic and not to indulge, not to increase conceitedness, and only in order to maintain my body, and prolong life, and to quench hunger, so that I can commit wholesome deeds to benefit myself and to benefit others...I will benefit by this food in prolonging my life, in leading a wholesome and peaceful life.

You can also consider and reflect upon this prayer during your meal. The fruits of your efforts can create a better attitude toward food, including the ability to overcome temptation, overindulgence, and unhealthy eating habits. One benefit of beginning any meal with a prayer is that it helps you to pause before eating.

Be Attentive. When we are attentive to the needs of others at the dinner table, we show them courtesy, compassion, and respect. Through small acts of mindfulness and thoughtfulness, such as anticipating when someone needs more food or drink, we become centered in the present moment.

If desired, silence can be incorporated into the meal. By maintaining silence we are less distracted and can be more fully aware of such things as how quickly we eat, how well we chew our food, what food we desire, and how much we eat.

Just as during meditation we don't fill up our lungs completely with each breath, we need to leave space in our stomachs when eating. This helps us establish moderate eating habits and, metaphorically, lets us transcend our self-limiting behaviors and overwhelming desires. By giving ourselves space—in our stomachs, in our lungs, and in our minds—we can know and experience that there is always room for expansion and growth in our lives.

End with a Blessing and Transmit Loving-Kindness. After the meal, sit silently and respectfully for a moment. Place your palms together over your heart center and say a loving-kindness blessing or grace for others:

May all beings be free from pain, hunger, and suffer-
ing. May all beings live long and be healthy. May all
beings receive physical nourishment, well-being, and
spiritual awareness through food. May all beings ex-
perience loving-kindness and serve others with compassion.

This lets you accomplish two things. First, you bless your food with loving-kindness. This gives your meal meaning and helps your body digest and receive full nourishment from food; it also reinforces spiritual consciousness and healthy eating habits. Second, you transmit loving-kindness to others—a step toward manifesting change in the world.

Should the reflection feel too long or cumbersome, try shortening it and putting it in your own words. Keep the essence of loving-kindness, and of food's purpose to yourself and others.

PRACTICE: NONATTACHMENT AND MODERATION

Savoring food with the senses offers a temporary worldly bliss. Eating food with spiritual awareness offers the potential of a more compassionate world and spiritual bliss. Through nonattachment and moderation we can appreciate and observe food's true meaning. This simple and elegant inner meal practice takes only moments and can be used before any meal or snack.

Training of any kind requires repetition, so remind yourself to pause and reflect on food's higher purpose at every meal. Do this inner meal practice until reflection at mealtime becomes a new habit—a process which usually takes one to three months, though you will feel the results as soon as you begin this practice.

As you continue on your road to self discovery, you may find that nonattachment and moderation liberate you from over-

whelming desire. This may let you step more securely onto the inner meal path.

The first part of this exercise is straightforward: pause before eating. Even if you've been conditioned to pick up the fork and dig in, pause for a moment to focus your inner awareness. Take a few seconds to observe the food and feel what it provides for you in terms of health and well-being. By focusing only on the higher meaning and value of food, you practice nonattachment from your emotional connection to it. Notice what draws your attention to the food before you—its look, its flavor, its scent. In your mind's eye, make a checklist of those qualities of food that increase your feelings of hunger and greed and desire. For example, you might think, "I am drawn to this food's juiciness," or "I am attracted to the crunchiness and richness of this food." Be patient as you do this, and allow yourself to note these qualities dispassionately—like a detective who is solving a mystery. Later, jot down these qualities in a notebook.

By permitting yourself to experience a "desire-free moment," you slowly break the bonds of attachment to food. If you have a desire or an impulse to eat immediately, just note that in your mind dispassionately, with a sense of nonattachment.

Second, make a point of starting with an empty plate. (If you are eating at a restaurant, it may be useful to ask for an extra plate.) Make it your job—and no one else's—to place just as much food on your plate as you think your body needs. If you want to put more on the plate, just note this desire in your thoughts: "I feel desire for food and want to put an extra helping on my plate." Even if you finish eating a plateful, take a second helping according to what you think your body needs. Try to be aware of when your body has enough nourishment. If you take only as much as you require, you'll avoid wasting food and overeating.

Third, recognize and be aware of your food choices. Know that you have complete freedom to pick the food that best serves you now. It may help to reflect on food's ultimate purpose—as the provider of your life energy and consciousness. By doing this, you bring moderation into your life and are less likely to abuse a particular food. You are also respecting your life and the value that food brings to it.

But what if you make a less than ideal food choice? Take responsibility for your choices, and know that while you might have fallen short of your ideal right now, you can make a better choice at the very next meal. In this way, moderation teaches us compassion for ourselves.

If you have a hard time feeling the importance of food's ultimate purpose, try to visualize what your life would be like if you didn't have enough food or didn't have the right food for good health. Eventually, you would suffer hunger, be unable to think properly, and become physically weak. All good things in life would lose their luster and become meaningless. Your existence would be consumed by trying to fill this one vital need. Keep in mind—this isn't supposed to make you feel sad or depressed or fearful—the purpose of this exercise is to allow you to feel the essence of food's ultimate purpose as giver of life and consciousness.

There are many benefits to practicing nonattachment and moderation at mealtime. It bolsters our intuition about what kinds of food we need. It improves digestion. It teaches patience. It lets us avoid wasting food. It gives us a more accurate sense of how much food we require for optimum health—no more and no less. Freedom of food choice brings true liberation from habit, and from such humble beginnings the soul takes wing.

5 – Holiness and Family

I am my beloved's,
and his desire is for me.
Come, my beloved,
let us go forth into the fields,
and lodge in the villages;
let us go out early to the vineyards,
and see whether the vines have budded,
whether the grape blossoms have opened
and the pomegranates are in bloom.
There I will give you my love.

—Song of Songs

It is a Friday night in Los Angeles. I've been invited to a Sabbath celebration, and unfortunately, I'm running late. A dense curtain of rain clogs traffic and makes the darkness appear even more deep and impenetrable. All the address numbers are swallowed in the shroud.

In truth, however, my anxiety stems not from the weather, but from the fact that I can't recall the last Sabbath I attended. I only know one person who will be there. I don't even remember a single prayer. I wonder if that's how the yeshiva students of Eastern Europe felt when they got invited to a stranger's home for a Sabbath or a holiday meal. At least, I muse, the yeshiva students *knew* the prayers.

Through fogged-up windows and the rhythmic splish-splash of windshield wipers I peer outside. I don't have a clue as to what the building looks like. Luckily, I nab the sole remaining parking space in front of the only structure showing any signs of life. Approaching the front door, I see the lit candles through the window. The ceremony has already begun.

Not wanting to interrupt, I stand under the eaves listening to the patter of raindrops. A few minutes later a woman with an umbrella walks up the driveway and asks whether I've come for the Sabbath. I nod, feeling a bit silly standing there in the rain. I follow her to the back of the building, where we enter.

Inside, I tiptoe into a room where the Sabbath candles burn without so much as a flicker. It's totally quiet as I take my seat on a small blue cushion among the fifteen meditators at the Zen Center of Los Angeles. I haven't been to many Sabbaths in my life, and surely never anything like this. I meditate for about twenty minutes until I hear the sound of a muffled bell.

Los Angeles Rabbi Don Singer, who also has the distinction of being a Zen master, begins by talking about the Sabbath, what it means, and even how it relates to Zen. Other participants share some ideas. One woman sings a song. Pages are handed out containing Hebrew prayers and some translations. The prayers are not said in rote fashion as I remember them from my childhood. Here, the rabbi pauses to explain the nuances of words and the history of the language. He weaves the riveting tale of his own boyhood pilgrimage to Israel with a Talmudic story about a Jewish mystic. There are questions. We sing. I have difficulty with the phonetic translations, but feel the joy of participating. Although I haven't spoken to a single person, I can sense the heart and spirit of this small gathering.

We move into another room where the *kiddush*, or sanctifying prayer, is said over wine. The words seem dimly familiar, like a forgotten child's rhyme remembered. Then, there is a prayer for bread. All of us take hold of two exquisitely braided loaves of challah to form a circle. I tear off a large nugget with delight. All our energy suddenly spills over, and we begin to chatter and eat chunks of bread like hungry schoolchildren at recess.

Perhaps most incredible of all, I realize I am no longer a stranger. This, I suddenly grasp, is the power of an ancient ritual written down thousands of years before. But on this night—indeed, on every Sabbath night—it lives, experienced joyously through a prayer, a song, a glass of wine, and a piece of challah.

The Jews are sometimes known as "people of the book" because their more than twenty-five-hundred-year-old Hebrew scriptures contain the wisdom of many books, including the Bible and a series of rabbinic writings such as the Talmud and midrash. The Torah, which consists of the five books of Moses, is alluded to as the "tree of life." That's because it is experienced by Jews as a living, breathing storehouse of God's love and wisdom.

The religion of the Jews brings its people into a covenant with a demanding, dominant, and powerful God who created heaven and Earth, man and woman, beasts and plants. Here, Earth is not anything like Hinduism's world of *maya*, or illusion. Neither is it like the Buddhist's world of impermanence and desire. Here, the Bible says that God recognized his work, and "God saw that it was good." So, while God is set apart from nature, His giving of life is an ultimate affirmative act of the divine. Earth's creations are to be embraced, relished, and cherished.

There is even a distant Pagan connection to the divine "Goddess," which reveals itself in Judaism's mystical tradition of the Kabbalah. Andrew Harvey, in *The Essential Mystics*, says that "the sacred feminine in Judaism is found in its sense of the sacredness of human life in all of its particulars when sanctified by prayer and the observation of sacred tradition: in eating, marriage, childbearing, and holy friendship as well as in prayer, contemplation, and ritual worship."

It is no wonder that the Hebrew scriptures draw upon a riveting narrative about creation in which food plays a significant role. A blissful Adam and Eve taste of the forbidden Tree of Knowledge and are forever exiled from the Garden of Eden. As in the Buddhist and Hindu traditions, the temptation of food reveals man's dual nature—his physical nature and human desires on the one hand, and his quest for spiritual development and the divine on the other. For Jews, however, the loss of bliss finds a worthy substitute in the search for meaning and holiness.

> *Rabbi Jacobs used to say:*
> *Better a single moment*
> *of awakening in this world*
> *than eternity in the world to come.*

—the *Pirke Avot* 6:11, "The Essential Mystics"

Finding Holiness and Meaning Through Food

For Jews, the inner meal path—as established in the ancient, daily practice of *kashrut*, or Jewish dietary laws—acts as a sacred conduit for awakening to meaning and holiness. These laws, found in both the Bible and the Talmud, are sometimes mistakenly thought to be about health. While kashrut may offer health benefits, its true purpose is clear: to make food *kadosh*, or holy, and to teach respect for life. It is through the observance of dietary laws that Jews hallow food and become a holy people.

The Bible requires that Jews imitate and follow God's own precepts, morals, and actions. The reason, plainly stated in Leviticus, is that "You shall be holy; for I the Lord your God am holy." Just as God blessed, hallowed and "rested from all his work" on the seventh day, so do the Jews rest on the Sabbath day. And, just as God tells which foods are clean and holy, so do Jews follow God's example by hallowing food.

This act of hallowing elevates food from the ordinary to the holy. Even more so, it raises all of life, including common, seemingly insignificant moments, onto hallowed ground. In *The Jewish Dietary Laws: Their Meaning For Our Time*, Rabbi Samuel Dresner writes that "in hallowing *we* become hallowed, in making our habits holy *we* become holy. A whole people becomes holy—'a kingdom of priests and a holy nation'; an entire nation set apart for His service. Judaism is a way of life, which encompasses the kitchen and the dining room as well as the Synagogue."

Beyond its role in the observance of dietary laws, food serves another key purpose: meals become a tangible remembrance of things past. Through an imaginative and interactive means of storytelling, food symbolizes Jewish history and brings it to life. Just as memories of my family's Sunday dinners are a cherished part of my personal story, a ritual meal of remembrance is a treasured part of the communal Jewish story.

Passover—A Meal of Remembrance

One celebration that symbolically uses food to evoke meaning, emotion, and poignancy is that of Passover. This spring festival commemorates the Jews' exodus from Egypt. The story of the Jews' slavery and subsequent flight to freedom is also significant for its biblical connection to Christianity and Islam. Christianity's Last Supper—itself a ritual Passover meal—tells its own story of remembrance, redemption, and communion through the use of bread and wine. Passover, with its universal theme of freedom, defines and keeps Judaism's values alive by extending a torch of remembrance from one generation to the next.

The festival centers on the *seder*, or Passover ritual meal. During the festival—which lasts for either seven or eight days depending on the religious tradition—families hold either one or two seder meals. The entire family reads from the Haggadah, a prayer book written especially for the Passover meal. To accommodate everyone—families, children, and Orthodox alike—Haggadoth vary in their use of language, tone, and emphasis. The story of Passover, as described in the Haggadah, lets family members experience the ordeals of the Jews as they prepared for and attained freedom from the pharaoh.

The seder ceremony includes special foods placed on a seder plate. These are tasted and explained at various times during the seder—with each food contributing meaning to the story. As such, the seder plate contains sprigs of parsley—or other leafy vegetables representing springtime—that are dipped in salt water to symbolize the tears of the slaves. Bitter herbs—often horseradish—recall the bitterness and pain of living in servitude. A coarse mixture of nuts and fruits—known as *charoset*—is reminiscent of the mortar Jews were forced to make into bricks while in bondage. A roasted hard-boiled egg reminds Jews of the ancient temple sacrifice offered on Passover. The egg also signifies—as it does for the Christian celebration of Easter—the transcendence of life beyond death.

Two other symbolic staples found at the Passover table include wine and *matzo*, or unleavened bread. Traditionally, a cup of wine is set on the table for the arrival of the prophet Elijah. Matzo reminds Jews of their escape to freedom, because in the haste to flee, there was no time for bread dough to rise. As a meal of remembrance, Passover brings the family together in a special way.

Daily Blessings and Mitzvah

In Judaism, spiritual growth depends on the personal effort and practice that one puts into studying the scriptures, performing good deeds, and praying. There is no free spiritual lunch, no sudden flash of enlightenment. Daily prayers and blessings, especially, form the mainstay of the work of hallowing foods. Neither are these blessings to be a felt as a rigid structure of beliefs. Instead, they are like holy threads that knit together the fabric of our daily human struggle.

Jewish blessings are wide and varied. In *The Jew in the Lotus*—a true story chronicling a pilgrimage to India by a group of religious Jews to meet the Dalai Lama—Rodger Kamenetz writes: "It seems our encounter with the Dalai Lama presented a unique challenge in the long history of Jewish blessings. Their delightful variety covered almost every situation. There is a blessing on seeing a rainbow or an extraordinarily beautiful person. On seeing fruit trees in bloom or for an assembly of more than six hundred thousand Jews...There is probably no extant blessing for a computer chip, but there is a blessing for pizza, fashioned from a blessing for bread." Kamenetz goes on to tell how, for the first time, the rabbis created a

Jewish prayer to "recognize the sacred in other religions."

The Jewish celebration of the Sabbath, for example, exemplifies the portable altar. With each weekly Sabbath meal, the common dinner table transforms into a beautifully decorated altar covered with slender candles, fine linens, fresh flowers, freshly baked bread, sweet wine, ornate table settings, and savory, nutritious food. Add to this the Sabbath's washing of hands and ritual blessings, and it becomes a holy offering to God.

The Sabbath meal also hallows the family and the community. Rabbi Don Singer once told me, "The only time food becomes good is when men and women come together in their wholeness." He was right.

Food is the magnet that pulls us home to our family and friends. It cultivates caring, love, compassion, and giving among those closest to us. It draws our attention to family and the values it stands for. It develops and deepens the bonds of friendship and community.

Not only is feeding the hungry part of Jewish tradition; it's woven into the fabric of Judaism by an inner meal practice known as a *mitzvah*, or a commandment from God to do good deeds. In mitzvah beats the spiritual heart of Judaism. To perform mitzvah— *mitzvoth* in the plural—is to exercise loving-kindness, compassion, giving, and service for others throughout the day. Inviting guests over for dinner, showing hospitality, feeding the hungry, and performing good deeds are not a matter of choice. God expects all this from us, and no less.

It's an old Jewish tradition to perform mitzvah by feeding the poor and inviting strangers to dinner on special holidays. In this sense, mitzvah is also a blessing—for it offers us comfort and joy by extending family to whoever happens to be a guest at our table.

Mitzvah makes the care of our neighbors a vital concern. The opportunity to perform mitzvah presents itself to us daily. Yet, how sad it is that in today's urban milieu, many of us fear helping others. To be asked for help by another is to raise hundreds of well-conditioned and habituated red flags in our mind. Some may be raised with good cause; many are not. To never help another, to never open to that possibility may ensure a certain kind of safety through insulation. But at what cost? How much of our own humanity is sacrificed when we close the door of a giving heart?

If you possess a well-developed cynical side that no longer believes what you do really matters, or if you are a person with the average amount of fear of the unknown, here is proof that your action, your loving-kindness, your good deed transmit hope and faith to others. Life matters because your mitzvah *makes* life matter.

Yet, while Judaism answers the questions about caring for our neighbors, it raises other important questions. While Jews hallow the life-affirming acts of creation, the Book of Genesis also states: "and let them have dominion over the fish of the sea, and over the birds of the air, and over the cattle, and over all the earth, and over every creeping thing that creeps upon the earth." In a master stroke, unique within religious history, man becomes an agent of God. As such, man's purpose is to shape the natural world as he deems fit. Earth and nature remain the domain of man.

This dominion sets in motion a two-edged sword—the eternal struggle between self interest and stewardship. All of Earth exists for man's sole use and pleasure, something to be celebrated and exalted. At the same time, the blue planet's care and well-being rest upon frail human shoulders as a sacred responsibility.

This presents a challenge for us as individuals and as members of the community. Now the question becomes: How do we act responsibly on behalf of Earth? How do we use our technology? How do we stop our wasteful habits?

According to the Bible, Jacob wrestled with God until the break of dawn when God said "'Your name shall no more be called Jacob, but Israel,' for you have striven with God and with men, and have prevailed." Jacob's name was changed because the word Israel means "to wrestle with God." Maybe the answer about how we will meet these challenges lies in our willingness, like Jacob's and Prince Arjuna's, to wrestle with our divine and human natures. And perhaps mitzvah has something to teach us about how to affirm life by accepting our responsibility as stewards of Earth and of all God's creations.

A Spiritual Meal Guideline

For Jews, meaning abounds wherever you happen to be. Or, whenever you happen to sit down to a meal or observe a holiday. Ingeniously, Judaism converts every home into a place of sacred worship, and every dinner table into a portable altar. The secret to creating a meal of observance and remembrance comes from finding the sacred meaning of food. What follows is one example of how you can experience the traditional Jewish practice of blessing and hallowing all aspects of your meal.

Wash the Hands. Jewish ritual cleansing echoes from history and the ancient rites performed by holy men who purified themselves at the temple altar before making a sacrificial offering. At the modern table, however, cleansing serves a very different function. Daniel Gordis, author of *God Was Not in the Fire*, writes that after pouring water over each hand, participants "recite a blessing, and then without speaking move back to their seat, recite a blessing over bread, and then begin to eat. It is a momentary ritual, without fanfare and without the pomp and circumstance of other religious events. But it is important. Like kashrut, it creates a brief silence, an opportunity to feel something."

Begin with a Prayer. The use of a *berakhah*, or blessing, is a constant staple at Jewish meals. As mentioned above, silence typically follows the cleansing of hands, after which a blessing is recited over the bread:

> *Blessed are You, Lord our God, Eternal One, Who brings forth bread from the earth.*

This blessing, in fact, precedes all meals because there is no minor or insignificant meal. Each morsel affirms the holiness and sanctity of life.

Enjoy Your Meal. Today, while many Jewish meals consist of vegetarian fare, the laws of kashrut permit the eating of meat that is *kosher*, or slaughtered and blessed in a special way that makes it suitable for consumption—a concept detailed in chapter 13.

Whatever food graces your table—from the traditional matzo ball soup and a chicken dish to a slice of apple strudel—every aspect of the meal should be savored and blessed. In addition, readings from the Torah, song, and lively discussion combine to give the traditional Jewish meal a truly inner meal dimension. Of course, you can choose to make your meal a mitzvah by inviting others to take part in hallowing it.

For those who include wine at the dinner table, the blessing over wine reads:

> *Blessed are You, Lord our God, Eternal One, Who creates fruit of the vine.*

End with a Blessing. Conclude your meal with a centering blessing, such as this Jewish prayer:

> *Blessed are You, Lord our God, Eternal One, Who grants us life, sustains us, and helps us reach this day.*

According to tradition, all knives are either covered up or removed from the table before singing the *Birkat Hamazon*, or grace, at the meal's end. This action serves to eliminate any possible representation of violence at what is a peaceful, harmonious, and sacred dinner.

PRACTICE: MITZVAH

There is something magical about mitzvah, and its practice can lead you to a hidden place within your soul—a gentle garden blossoming with grace and wonderment. For their meaning to be fulfilled, these deeds must be performed joyously, from the heart. Never is mitzvah to be felt or experienced as a burden or unwanted obligation.

There are different kinds of mitzvah. Some play a role in ritual, such as lighting candles or cleaning out leavened bread from the house as required during the Passover holiday. Others play a role in service to the community, such as donating time to feed the poor or offering food to a charitable organization. Practicing mitzvah puts you firmly on the road to self-discovery. Have you performed mitzvah today? If not, there's no better time than the present.

As you perform your mitzvah—or mitzvoth—give it or them much thought. Think about what service, charity, or good deed you want to perform with a joyful heart. Since this book is about the *art of the inner meal,* you might invite a single or elderly neighbor over for dinner. Ask that hungry person on the corner what he or she needs to eat. Drop off excess canned goods at a nearby soup kitchen. Volunteer to deliver food to the hungry through a worthwhile organization. Or, perform your mitzvah like a pot luck—spontaneously as the need arises.

Inherent in mitzvah is a sense of uncertainty. This uncertainty and unknowing bring freedom and spontaneity to your mitzvah. With uncertainty there are no limits placed on it. The surprise, joy, and direction of your mitzvah are a unique, living expression of your kindness to others. Allow yourself to perform mitzvah with uncertainty. This enables you to open yourself up fully to the experience, and to the complete range of possibilities that giving and receiving create.

Remember, your intent to give mitzvah is return enough. If someone doesn't thank you or give you the positive response you want, this does not lessen your act of kindness. But chances are your good deed will be appreciated.

Mitzvah costs us nothing but the realization that all of us possess common needs and concerns. Ask yourself: "What would a day with mitzvah be like? How would it change my own life and the life of others?" Once you perform mitzvah, you may wonder how you went so long without it in your life.

The inner meal practice of mitzvah offers many enduring benefits. It fosters living life in the present moment, because we never know how or when the opportunity to do a good deed will arise. It encourages improvement of our communities and neighborhoods. It promotes giving and feeds the hungry. It makes every day meaningful. And, not least of all, mitzvah gives each of us the feeling that we've made a difference and accomplished something very important—and we have.

6 - Community and Communion

Take me with you on this journey
Where the boundaries of time are now tossed
In cathedrals of the forest
In the words of the tongues now lost

Find the answers, ask the questions
Find the roots of an ancient tree
Take me dancing, take me singing
I'll ride on till the moon meets the sea

—Loreena McKennitt, lyrics from "Night Ride
Across the Caucasus"

A little over two thousand years ago, a man stepped out of the
wilderness filled with the message and the spirit of God. Though
not much is known about the life of Jesus, his teachings endure
today in all corners of the world. Food was very important to Jesus,
and he used it to differentiate his teachings from what had come
before.

Many scholars believe—as supported by the findings of the
Dead Sea Scrolls—that Jesus was well-versed in the ideas of the

Essenes. The Essenes, a Jewish sect of which John the Baptist was probably a member, were greatly influenced by the ideas of the Pythagorean societies of Alexandria. This fact was reported by Josephus, a Jewish historian who lived among the Essenes. This means that besides practicing the traditional Jewish rituals of Sabbath, kashrut, and mitzvah, the Essenes apparently practiced many Greek-inspired customs like vegetarianism and ritual purification through baptism.

We all respond to the pressures and forces of society in different ways. Huston Smith, in his well-known standard *The World's Religions*, describes the core controversies swirling around the beleaguered Judaism of Jesus' era. Among the major sects were the Sadducees, Jews who "accommodated themselves to Hellenistic culture and Roman rule." The Pharisees revered charity and the laws of holiness as a way to make Judaism "a beachhead of holiness in human history." The Essenes believed that the world was corrupt and "so they dropped out...[and] devoted themselves to lives of disciplined piety."

Jesus, like the Pharisees, practiced both charity and mitzvah. But he differed in one respect: he felt that God's compassion was more important than adhering to holy food codes that formed unholy distinctions between people. Wasn't it better to make all foods clean and let everyone come together at the same table— regardless of dietary laws and religious beliefs—without differences and judgment?

When Jesus was asked—as described in Mark's Gospel—why his disciples did not follow tradition and wash their hands before eating, he replied that "there is nothing outside a man which by going into him can defile him; but the things which come out of a man are what defile him." In this way, Jesus made a clean break with Jewish dietary laws, and the knife that made the precisionlike cut was compassion.

Once Jesus cast his lot in this direction, writes Huston Smith, "he parleyed with tax collectors, dined with outcasts and sinners, socialized with prostitutes, and healed on the sabbath when compassion prompted doing so. This made him a social prophet, challenging the boundaries of the existing order and advocating an alternative vision of the human community."

It was out of compassion that Jesus performed several of his food-related miracles, such as turning a few loaves of bread and a few fish into enough food to feed thousands. Jesus commingled charity and compassion in a social setting. Even today, this is a powerful combination, and the evangelical energy of Jesus' actions and ideas lives on in the Christian ideals of charitable service within the community—ideals attainable through the path of the inner meal. As if to confirm this, a Benedictine monk once told me with a wink and a smile, "The two things that Jesus does in the New Testament are to eat and heal."

The early Christian monastic movement was one of the first to recognize and strengthen this link between community and Christianity. Basil the Great—a fourth-century monk—helped realize the social potential of Jesus' vision. Since he believed that Jesus' teachings and the Bible provided all the necessary answers about how to live communally, he directed the activities of monks toward meeting society's needs. Eventually, the Church accepted the value of the monastic example of how to live a Christian life within a close-knit community—one in which feeding others plays a major part.

A Morning Call

It is a Tuesday morning when I get a frantic call from Claire, the coordinator at the local meals-on-wheels. It turns out that she badly needs a rider for the Blue Route. Usually, I get called Sunday or Monday, but a "regular" has dropped out at the last minute. I'm one of the substitutes on her list. I'm glad she called me, because it's an opportunity to visit the Blue Route people again. Arriving at the kitchen at around 11:30 A.M., I sign in and put on a name tag that identifies me as a meals-on-wheels volunteer. It's a joy to see Claire, a short, gray-haired dynamo who has given service to her community for many years. Sometimes I think of asking her why she has done this for so long, but the answer is obvious: she loves what she's doing.

Today I'm riding along with Bob, who is eight years retired from a job with the Los Angeles school district. This is Bob's regular route, and he knows it by heart. Our second stop is at a building for seniors. I hop out of Bob's truck, open an insulated container, and cradle four meals in my arms: three regular, one diabetic. Bob handles the hot meals.

I also carry cards with statistics on each recipient: age, medical condition, and the date started on the meals-on-wheels program. As we walk down a drab hallway to our next delivery, something on a card catches my eye. It's the word *artist*, which is interesting, since the cards don't usually mention any personal information other than medical.

We tap gently on the door. A diminutive lady greets us, smiling. Now I remember the last time I was here. Her husband had fallen out of his wheelchair onto the living room floor, and she was upset, unable to lift him. Today he is in bed. We set the hot and cold meals on a round table.

I ask, "Is your husband an artist?"

Her eyes widen. "How did you know that?" she says with great surprise.

"It was written on his card," I say, spying a painting on the wall.

"This is one of his," she says proudly.

We move in for a closer look. It's an oil painting, a stunning, detailed depiction of wooden Korean battleships from three hundred years ago engaged in a battle upon a roiling, tumultuous sea. I assume it's a famous battle, but do not ask.

It's beautiful," echo Bob and I. As we leave, I walk past the bedroom and glance momentarily at the ninety-year-old man who painted this picture almost two decades ago. Resting on his side, he watches us, attention riveted. The memories hanging on the walls, the photos of loved one on the mantels—these are some of the things we care about when we grow old. But there is more.

I recall the simple questions that Jack Kornfield asks of us in *A Path with Heart*:

> *In the stress and complexity of our lives, we may forget our deepest intentions. But when people come to the end of their life and look back, the questions that they most often ask are seldom, "How much is in my bank account?" or "How many books did I write" or "What did I build?" or the like. If you have the privilege of being with a person who is aware at the time of his or her death, you find the questions such a person asks are very simple: "Did I love well?" "Did I live fully?" "Did I learn to let go?"*

Most of the community of people Bob and I deliver meals to are elderly. The majority live alone, having lost their husband or wife along the way. Many are in their late eighties and early nineties. Josephine is like that. Her card tells me that she is ninety-one years old, afflicted with arthritis, uses a walker, and suffers constant pain.

The Spanish-style house, which incorporates graceful stucco archways common to homes built here in the 1920s, is immaculately maintained. Bob and I knock, and the unlocked door hinges open. We call out. A feeble but clear-toned voice answers and tells us to enter. The light inside is dim. I set the meal down and turn toward the darkness of the living room. Josephine sits perched on the edge of a love seat, one hand anchored to a metallic walker. She asks my name so she will remember it the next time, and we share some small talk about the weather, how she likes her meals—that kind of thing.

When we prepare to leave, Josephine rises with difficulty, a look of arthritic pain on her face. I want to tell her it's unnecessary, but don't. Ever so slowly, she shuffles over to the open door until we say good-bye. In the light, her clear, liquid blue eyes sparkle like sapphires. We'd like to talk some more, Bob explains, but others are expecting us.

We slowly close the front door behind us. The sun remains high in the cloudless sky. We walk past a large, thick-trunked tree with white bark split with age. It was probably planted when the house was built. There's a sense of continuity, a sense of community here. Right now, in a small way, I am a part of it, part of its spirit. And that is all that matters.

Finding Communion Through Food

Spirit, in the Christian sense, also has a lot to do with Jesus' directions regarding bread and wine at The Last Supper. Here is basis of a sacred inner meal practice, one in which bread and wine transmute into the blood and flesh of the Christ. Food serves as a holy passage through which Jesus' disciples experience God's forgiveness and love. For some Christians this ritual transmutation is literal, while for others it is symbolic. Either way, food transforms from the material and physical into pure spirit. Through the inner meal practice of taking communion, one receives not physical nourishment so much as the spiritual essence of God. In this way God is always available, always present.

Jesus, much like the Buddha, used his own life to show the frailty, weakness, and suffering of human beings. Unlike the Buddhists, however, Christians believe Jesus suffered and sacrificed and died to atone for all human sin. For them, the Holy Communion reaffirms this fact. Taking communion is to surrender to the Spirit of God, to take Christ into oneself, or, as Saint Paul says, to be "in Christ." As Father Thomas Keating writes in *Open Mind, Open Heart,* "Faith is opening and surrendering to God. The spiritual journey does not require going anywhere because God is already with us and in us." And neither is this surrender a solitary act, for it is just as much a communion with others.

It is a weekday morning, and I have driven up the Pacific coastline to Mount Calvary Monastery. The monastery is tucked in the mountains, some 1,250 feet above the city of Santa Barbara. I sit on a sun-bleached porch just outside the chapel, looking at the faraway, meandering coastline. The air is still and quiet, save the chirping of birds and the occasional clang of pots coming from the monastery kitchen. It is almost twelve o'clock and time for the daily communion to begin.

We start by singing. I don't know any of the hymns, but I share a prayer book with someone and do the best I can. Later, each of the five Benedictine monks who are present takes a turn expressing his thoughts and feelings about the life of Saint Teresa of Ávila. It's a sublime moment, as each Brother speaks of this extraordinary woman and sixteenth-century founder of many religious houses, and what she means to them. The personalities of the monks reveal themselves through this spontaneous exercise. There are moments when we laugh, moments when we choke up with emotion. Moments of silence. Together, we read some of Saint Teresa's prayers. Finally, we rise and form a circle in preparation for communion. We sing, hold hands, say, "May peace be with you" to one another, and then take communion one by one. When the Eucharist is complete, we walk no more than ten steps to the dining room for lunch. The spirit among us is featherlike. After grace, spoken by Brother Lawrence, we form a line for food.

At the time of the Last Supper, the sacrament of communion was not separate from the meal. For many years that tradition carried on, and I can understand why. Eating after a holy communion reminds us that all food is sacred. It allows the personal experience of God to be part of a shared communion with others. Every time we eat with others, we commune with them.

I am reminded of a recent visit with Brother Roy Parker, Order of the Holy Cross (O.H.C.), a thin, soft-spoken monk who lives at Mount Calvary, to talk about food, spirituality, and the larger meaning of communion. After arriving, I watch as Brother Roy prepares the dough for the multigrain bread that he bakes for the monks and visitors. After a few minutes, he sets the dough aside to let it rise, and I offer to help him wash and clean the utensils. We do this silently, and when finished, sit on stools at a tall island of weathered wooden butcher block.

The talk gets around to what makes his homemade bread—or should I say "monastery-made"?—bread so special. I've had the pleasure of eating it, and it is spectacular, a virtual meal in itself. Brother Roy explains that even when cooking food, "you just have to have the spirit in communion with what you're doing, and the ingredients will take care or themselves." The art of the inner meal means being in communion with all aspects of food, and of life. By expanding our personal concept and practice of communion we make every meal—from preparation to cleanup—joyous and special.

Prayer and Fasting

Food connects to the Spirit in yet another way for the Christian tradition—through renunciation, which is achieved by sacred prayer and fasting. It is in the Bible's story of Jesus' forty days and nights in the desert wilderness, for example, that renunciation takes on special meaning. A hungry Jesus, having fasted for the entire time, is tempted to eat by the devil, who asks him to turn stones into loaves of bread. Instead of giving in, Jesus resists by quoting the Bible:

> *Man shall not live by bread alone, but by every word that proceeds from the mouth of God.*

As in communion, here is a clear victory of spirit over flesh. This story teaches us that, to the extent to that we can suppress our physical appetite, we can be nourished and strengthened instead by the spiritual meal. Fasting and prayer, according to Jesus, create such a powerful union that they are capable even of casting out the devil.

This practice of uniting prayer and fasting was used early on by the Christian monks who lived in Egypt during the second and third centuries. In the ascetic tradition, they lived in poverty and spent their days fasting—all the while nourishing their spirit by reciting scriptural passages. Looked at another way, doesn't renunciation diminish the ego and make room for God and the Spirit? Doesn't it give us the greater spiritual capacity we need to be more charitable toward others? The more we use the inner meal practice of fasting and prayer to restrict food—a practice detailed in chapter 12—the less likely we are to worship food, become obsessed by it, or let it become a stumbling block to providing charity for others. This same idea echoes through the Bible, and Corinthians tells us that the mistake made by some is to "eat food as really offered to an idol; and their conscience, being weak, is defiled. Food will not commend us to God. We are no worse off if we do not eat, and no better off if we do."

Think of the scales of justice. On one scale are desire and selfishness; balanced on the other scale are renunciation and charity, or selflessness. This is the Buddhist struggle between excess and abstinence all over again. There are numerous examples of extreme renunciation throughout Christian history. While giving up something as necessary for survival as food makes a powerful statement, most biblical fasting takes the middle road and is restricted to a day or less. Renouncing food reminds us that while we have a choice in the matter, others may not. In this way, charity becomes yet another way to navigate the inner meal path.

A Spiritual Meal Guideline

Historically, Christians experienced the Holy Communion in a home-based setting. Today, many capture this ritual's embracing spirit through a meal of communion with family and friends. What follows are suggestions to accessing the essence of such a meal. Whatever guidelines you decide to use, a meal of communion gives voice to your love of God and community.

Again, note the similarity in form and substance between this meal of communion and the patterns of spiritual meals in other traditions. Use these similarities to reinforce your spiritual meal practices.

Begin with a Prayer. Jesus made the decision regarding food, as did the Buddha before him, to take a compassionate course in terms of what one should eat. Because all foods are "clean" and proper in the Christian tradition, what's most important is *how* we approach food and others—through love as expressed in our thoughts, words, and actions. One way to begin your meal of communion is with a centering prayer, such as the Lord's Prayer, to invoke a divine presence:

> *Our Father (Mother) who art in Heaven, hallowed be thy name. Thy Kingdom come, thy will be done on Earth as it is in Heaven. Give us this day our daily bread and forgive us our trespasses, as we forgive those who trespass against us. And lead us not into temptation, but deliver us from evil, for Thine is the Kingdom and the power and the glory. For ever and ever. Amen.*

Share Stories and Communion. A further sense of unity can be created through the ancient Christian prayer practice of *Lectio Divina*, or "divine reading"—which is detailed in chapter 8. Use Lectio Divina to recite your favorite passages from the Bible, the Psalms, or other spiritual works.

This shared experience creates an atmosphere of compassionate listening and prepares everyone for the communion. As the focus of the gathering turns toward what it means to sacrifice, to sin, and to forgive, distribute bread and wine. After taking Holy Communion, those present may choose to break into smaller groups for song or prayer.

Enjoy Your Meal. Before eating, give thanks by reciting grace with words such as:

> *Our Father (Mother)... Bless us, Lord, and these gifts which we are about to receive from Thy bounty. Through Christ our Lord. Amen.*

In the spirit of communion, make a point of inviting to the meal someone who would benefit from the Christian ideals of love, compassion, forgiveness, charity, and hospitality. As you eat, savor God's bounty of food, but try not to overindulge or be obsessed by it. Remember that food, like communion, can be a vehicle for spiritual transmutation and transcendence.

End with a Blessing. Conclude this special meal by reciting a short blessing of grace, such as:

> *We give thanks, Lord, for all Thy benefits, Who lives and reigns the world without end. Amen.*

Sharing a moment of silence offers another meaningful way to bring the meal to a close. Use the silence to reflect upon a group prayer, an intention, or a vow—such as praying for the hungry or making a commitment to feed a hungry person during the week.

Or use the silence to perform an "Examen of Conscience." This is a method—explained in chapter 11—that we can use to examine our day's actions, determine if we have been hurtful or helpful to others, and ask for forgiveness.

PRACTICE: COMMUNITY AND SERVICE

It is easy to think that helping to feed and care for the community is not our responsibility. That's what government is for, isn't it? That's what our taxes are paying for, aren't they? Well, yes and no. There may always be a need for government assistance. Too many people fall through an imperfect and fragmented safety net. That's why we need to find out exactly who this "community" is that needs caring for.

Community exists much like the many thousands of unique strands of thread woven together to form protective clothing. Each of us is like a single thread in that fabric. A single strand, however, can't cover us, can't shield us from the sun, can't protect us from the cold.

This inner meal practice is really one of communion, for

it explores—and exposes—how we intermingle and meld our separate lives and dreams with those of others. It is through the quality and nature of our combined compassion, vision, and charitable service that we fashion the fabric of our community-communion.

Close your eyes and take a deep breath. Reflect for a moment about the relationship of your own thread of life to the whole. Where do you intersect with the rest of your community? Some threads may not be important to you and so you don't notice them. Yet they, too, are part of your community's fabric. Try to let yourself see those other threads.

Which ones help center your community? What ones nourish its peace and serenity? Which burst with energy? Do any threaten to fray or tear its fabric? You may witness this in terms of people, institutions, or ideas. As you witness, do so without a sense of righteousness and judgment. Instead, simply witness with the healing compassion practiced by Jesus and Buddha.

All the connections and threads will not be apparent immediately. If you become aware of just one new, small section of your community's fabric, then you have taken an important step. As you witness your community through reflection, you may find its fabric is frayed or torn apart, and that it needs fixing.

Now, the reflection becomes one of inquiry. How can you help make the necessary repairs? How can your efforts make a difference? How can you help realize your vision of how your community can unfold?

Make a list of the ways your community's fabric needs mending. Then, commit to a course of action by choosing to look to one or more of the needs that you've identified. Also, know that you needn't do this alone. Include friends and family in gaining a consensus about how to serve the community.

What sometimes stops us from action is the thought that the fabric is just too large. Well, no one expects you to change the world. Remember, this is your community you're looking at. It starts with your front yard, your block, your street, your lonely neighbor, your hungry beggar. At your own doorstep is as good a place to start as any. Any positive service, even if it impacts just one person, creates ripples that benefit us all.

There are a great many benefits to reflecting on community and service. We find that we are not powerless. We learn that caring for the community also means caring for ourselves. The Christian ideal of charitable community service engages our passion, makes us feel alive, and connects us with the divine. We become a living example of the Christian belief that the divisions between the rich and poor, and the haves and have-nots, are overcome with love and compassion. Through the inner meal practice of serving others, we connect to our responsibility and role in helping to maintain a caring community that addresses the needs of all.

7 – Surrender, Prayer, and Charity

*A certain person came to the Friend's
door and knocked.
"Who's there?"
"It's me."
The Friend answered, "Go away. There's
no place for raw meat at this table."
The individual went wandering for a year.
Nothing but the thirst of separation can
change hypocrisy and ego. The person
returned completely cooked, walked up
and down in front of the Friend's home,
gently knocked.
"Who is it?"
"You."
"Please come in, my Self. There's no place
in this house for two."*

— Rumi (Sufi poet), "The World's Wisdom"

The clouds hang thick, dark, and low in the early night sky. I carry
two thermos bottles from my cottage to the monastery kitchen. The
cottage contains no stove, and I must boil water for my tea and hot
drinks. The monks chant at 6 P.M. each evening, and I take care to

leave before then, so as not to disturb them. When I step back outside, the air turns suddenly cool. I feel the sprinkle of moisture that comes before rain. Soon it is dark. Inside the cottage, the patter of rain grows into a loud, persistent hiss. This rain, I think, expresses the surrender of the Earth—to heat, to dryness, to thirst, and to hunger. If only we could all surrender like this.

Surrender also has a lot to do with the essence of the word *Islam*, whose roots of *Silm* and *Salam* not only mean "peace," but convey the idea of surrender as well. This surrender is the giving up of oneself to live in peace—with God, with the community, and with oneself.

It was in the late sixth century, around 570, that Muhammad— "the praised one"—was born in Mecca, a thriving city located less than fifty miles from the Red Sea. He became the first person to bring the people of Arabia a holy scripture of their own—the Qur'an— in their native language of Arabic. What these scriptures have to say about food and giving connects, in many ways, to the ancient Arab traditions and the trials that Arabia faced leading up to the time of Muhammad.

While the Quraysh tribe that Muhammad was born into no longer lived a nomadic life, the function of tribe was still critical for personal and family survival. One's tribe acted as a safety net in hard times and as protection from other aggressive tribes and clans. By necessity, the tribal unit thrived by being both harsh and democratic. While survival of the fittest was the unwritten rule, food and spoils of war, for example, were shared among all. Traditionally, food was offered freely, in the knowledge that the favor might need to be reciprocated in times of scarcity.

As some Quraysh settled in Mecca and became successful merchants, however, they did not freely share of their wealth according to nomadic tradition. Muhammad's clan was among the poorer ones, and, having been twice orphaned, he acutely felt the pain of deprivation. Muhammad always championed equality and giving, and even before he received the Qur'an he often took solitary retreats during which he prayed and fed the poor.

In fact, of all the paths Muhammad could have chosen to proclaim his faith, the one that he embraced was the inner meal. After receiving God's Word, Muhammad preached quietly, only to those he trusted. When the time finally came to make a declaration to his entire clan, he did so over a meal—and it was one brimming with hidden meaning. Karen Armstrong, in *Muhammad: A Biography of the Prophet*, writes that "he went ahead and invited the forty leading men of Hashim to a modest meal. The meager repast was a message in itself: Muhammad had become very critical of the ostentatious hospitality that had become traditional among the Arabs as a display of power and confidence: He felt it smacked of the old presumption." Like the Buddha, Jesus, and others before him, Muhammad upset social convention in favor of what he believed was a more inspired and just way of living.

Islam's five pillars include a declaration of faith, prayer, the giving of alms, fasting, and pilgrimage. Together, these principles are designed to guide Muslims toward, as is written in the Qur'an, "the straight way. The way of those on whom Thou has bestowed Thy Grace."

Islam differs from other religions in that it specifically describes God's laws of how to live in the community, how much charity to give, and other practical aspects of living. Many food regulations and practices are found in the Hadith books—a collection of traditional guidelines containing a record of Muhammad's personal practices and sayings, as well as the consensus of scholars on what is proper.

For this reason, it's important for Muslims to know exactly which foods are considered to be *halal*, or lawful, and which foods are considered to be *haram*, which means "forbidden" or "unlawful"—concepts covered in greater detail in chapter 13. In this way, daily life becomes a direct means of showing faith in God and doing God's will—ideals clearly attainable through food.

The Value of Surrender

Muslims believe the Qur'an is neither interpretation nor commentary, but the direct, divine word of God's will as he revealed it to Muhammad. To surrender to God's presence, Muslims show reverence by invoking God's name before eating. Muslims also pray several times a day—and many of their prayers, even many daily actions, start with words that mean "In the name of God, who is most gracious and most merciful." In the larger sense, this allows them to "begin" almost any action "in the name of God" or with God in mind.

This powerful intention is recited often—whether boiling a pot of tea, preparing a meal, driving to the market, or getting ready to do almost anything. Consider this for a moment: Isn't this really a gentle, peaceful way of surrendering the outcome of our actions to God? Here is a way of letting go of our need for worldly control. After all, surrender to God is the cornerstone of faith.

The word *surrender* isn't fondly and commonly used these days. To think about surrender is to imagine the beaten, defeated faces of losers of wars. You won't see the word *surrender* in a corporate mission statement. You won't hear it spoken in politics, except maybe negatively. You won't hear sports teams utter a syllable of it. You won't find it in too many diet books. You probably won't or hear or feel it in too many families and relationships. My dictionary says that it means: "1. To give up control or possession of to another on demand or under compulsion. 2. To give (oneself) over, as to an emotion." Then again, we're talking about peaceful surrender, not forceful surrender.

Sometimes it helps to think about something in terms of its opposite. If surrender is such a bad thing, then the opposite of it must be good. But what if we always had to conquer, always had to win, always had to fear losing? To live like this is like strapping yourself into a straitjacket, with no room to move or ever change your mind—even if it's in your best interests to do so. To live like this is to allow no space for the thoughts and ideas of others, and, ultimately, no space for a mutually satisfying relationship.

The Qur'an promotes a life where surrender to God and giving to others are highly valued. *Sura*, or chapter, 89 speaks of a lack of surrender of those who "honor not the orphans. Nor do you encourage one another to feed the poor." This can also be interpreted to mean we all need to feed the emotionally orphaned and hungry part of ourselves.

Surrender or Submission?

It's easy to mistake surrender with submission, and it's the subtle difference between these two ideas that gives surrender a special place along the inner meal path. To submit to anything is to allow yourself to be subjected to the authority of another without your permission, control, will, or judgment. Surrender, on the other hand, can be experienced as a process of faith, and in this sense is actually a choice. By choosing to surrender we may actually be gaining—not losing—greater freedom, control, and access to deeper parts of ourselves.

Have you ever submitted to a diet? When you submit to another's diet you give up the most important part of yourself— your compassionate and knowing inner self. Some people stick to a diet whatever the consequences, even if it results in illness. We may think we are "in control," but actually we are passively relinquishing our control to something outside ourselves. Submitting to a rigid eating regimen to gain a specific result, for example, has the effect of reducing your body to a machine. But we are more than that. By submitting blindly we may automatically exclude a whole range of options.

On the other hand, by surrendering inwardly we open ourselves up to new and possibly unexplored territory. Now, try surrendering to that same diet, and the experience will be totally different. To surrender is to be alert and alive to the shifting sands of your whole inner landscape. This means you will experience the diet as a process, as a guideline to accomplish something, not merely as an end result. We do not lose ourselves by surrender, as we might fear. Rather, we gain insight, knowledge, and experience about our personal inner meal.

Sufi mystic Inayat Khan, in his classic work *The Gayan*, tells us something about the meaning of surrender in the personal realm:

The difference between war and peace
is that war is using sword against another
and peace is using sword toward oneself.
Fight against the enemy means war.
Fight against oneself means peace.

Surrendering in peace is something worked at slowly, over time. It is something that each of us, individually, learns how to do in our own way. This is also how we surrender to the inner meal.

Transformation Through Fasting, Charity, and Moderation

It is an uncommonly stormy morning in Southern California on this, the final and climactic day of Ramadan. More than ten thousand people overcome the elements and the morning traffic jams to cram into an immense hangar at a U.S. Marine base, where they pray and hear a sermon. All face toward the ancient city of Mecca, with feet, hands, knees, and foreheads touching the ground. The words "Allaahu Akbar Allaahu Akbar"—meaning "God is Greatest God is Greatest"—echo under the cavernous roof. In this gesture, Muslims share a collective sense of surrender and humility toward God. They also feel the collective bond that comes from a month of shared fasting and self-restraint.

The Ramadan month bestows togetherness in other ways, such as through shared meals—when groups meet after sunset to break their fast. Always, there is the constant sense of food's ultimate purpose and the sharing with others that it affords. Traditionally, these fasts are broken with dates, a food that Muhammad himself used to break the Ramadan fast. Could it be, I wonder, that Muhammad did this as a sign—to help us realize how sweet life is when we have the blessings of food to nourish ourselves and others? I like to think it is entirely possible.

Muslims believe that those who earnestly do without food during Ramadan attain rewards that stay with them throughout the year. For example, those who invite the hungry to break the fast, who sincerely perform their prayers, and who pass a night awake during Ramadan's last ten days are rewarded with forgiveness of past mistakes, peace of mind, and blessings.

The inner meal practice of fasting—one of Islam's five pillars—also encourages inner transformation. For Muslims, the fasting undertaken during the holy month of Ramadan holds special significance. Throughout this holy holiday Muslims recite the Qur'an from beginning to end, and each day they read aloud from its suras.

Ramadan uses the spiritual practice of fasting and prayer to test the will power, and to channel energy and awareness into the spiritual realm. The daily fast extends from sunrise to sunset, and during this time followers do not drink liquids or solid food. Nothing, not even smoke, passes their lips. They must even abstain from any impure thoughts or sex.

As Jesus showed, fasting and prayer are a potent consciousness-raising combination. And yet, does not Ramadan serve the spirit and the body in equal measure? In truth, it is not possible to fulfill the needs of one without the other. Without the physical body, we could not contain the soul and fulfill its purpose.

When at last the Ramadan fast concludes, it is celebrated on the thirtieth and final day with the fast-breaking feast of *Eid*, which means "to rejoice and be happy." This daylong celebration brings the community members together again with a renewed sense of meaning. Together, they have endured a fast and recited the Qur'an. At another level, Ramadan is living proof that compassion and strength are necessary to surrender. In this sacred way are we able to sustain one another and our inner selves.

Because transforming the inner self is only part of our work, Islam uses charity—another of its five pillars—to transform the community at large. Why charity? When the wealthy give to the poor, they are reminded that others are less fortunate. In this way, they do good deeds, share their happiness, improve society and the economy by reducing the burden of the poor, and follow God's will.

This annual charity, normally 2.5% of one's assets, is distributed to the poor according to the Qur'an, and the recipients needn't be Muslim. This form of charity often finds its way to poor relatives, deserving neighbors, and worthwhile community and city projects.

Muhammad, just like the Buddha, discovered the importance of moderation through an experience with food. This happened during a supreme vision—called the Night Journey—when Muhammad traveled at midnight to Jerusalem and ascended to God's throne. With the Bible's great prophets in attendance, Muhammad was offered three goblets from which to drink. One contained water, another milk, and another wine. By choosing milk, Muhammad symbolically chose the middle road of moderation between abstinence and excess.

To know the middle road requires personal initiative and practiced activity, because, says the Qur'an, "never will God change the condition of a people until they change their inner selves." Isn't this another way of saying that we need to surrender to inner change? And as so often happens on the road to self-discovery, we end up at the place where we started—only to begin our journey once again.

A Spiritual Meal Guideline

The Islamic meal is steeped in a long tradition that unites prayer and hospitality at mealtime. The suggestions that follow create a meal seasoned with healthful eating habits.

Wash the Hands. The Muslim practice of ablution—ritual purification through washing the face, hands, and feet—is a prerequisite before prayer and mealtime. Besides cleansing the body, ablution also purifies the spirit in preparation for food.

Begin with a Prayer. Traditionally, Muslims conduct "regular" prayers five times each day. These are conducted once before sunrise, three times during the day, and once before sunset. Regular prayers are highly ritualized and consist of several distinct movements.

A mealtime prayer like the following reminds us that food comes from the divine source:

O' Thou, sustainer of our bodies, hearts, and spirits—
bless all that we receive in thankfulness. Amin.
—Sufi Order of the West

Honor God's Will. Every meal contains the potential to express God's will regarding prayer, feeding others, and eating lawful and allowable foods to encourage good personal health. This also means controlling food intake, not wasting food, and understanding that at the spiritual level we are what we eat. Interestingly, the ancient Muslim practice of eating with the hands—a practice still used in some cultures—originated in the belief that the hands secrete a substance that aids in digestion.

All lawful foods—including certain meats—are acceptable at a Muslim dinner table. By adhering to food laws and taking responsibility for what we eat, we honor the will of God and those we love.

End with a Blessing. To show gratefulness to God for the food on your table, end your meal by saying grace.

PRACTICE: SURRENDERING

For some, surrendering may be one of the hardest paths to take. This road to self-discovery contains many bends and surprises. Yet, by venturing onto this path we can witness the dawn of our faith. If you are unsure, tread slowly. After all, isn't this how we trek up even the highest mountain—one small step at a time?

The idea of surrendering can be scary and difficult. But here's another way to view it: all you're really doing is developing faith. To surrender with peace means allowing yourself to enter a place with unbounded potential—where you don't know all the answers or the outcome.

Imagine for a moment that you are about to plan a very special dinner party. What kinds of feelings arise? What are your concerns? Are you worried that the food won't turn out just perfectly? Are you in a competition to outdo someone else with a more extravagant party? Or maybe you're worried that everyone will arrive late. Or that the music you have planned won't set the right mood. The list goes on and on. We've probably all experienced these fears and thoughts at one time or another.

Write down all your feelings, fears, hopes, and expectations regarding this dinner party. Putting them on paper makes it easy for you to reflect on them and think about why they matter.

Imagine what would happen if you decided not to measure the party's success or failure by how the food turned out, who showed up, or a hundred other things. Instead, what if you simply allowed yourself to surrender to the uncertainty of the moment? What if your only purpose was to be with people you knew and cared about? In this way you actually give up your fears and surrender to faith.

Many of us have a difficult time embracing faith, thinking that it means we are weak, irrational, or not in control. On the contrary, it means we are no longer relegated to being winners or losers. It lets us feel our greater connection to the oneness of the divine plan in which we all are winners by serving the will of God.

Write down your intent to surrender to faith, to feed others, and to provide a time and a place for people to share their stories in a meaningful way. No two dinners are alike. Whether you eat alone, or with the same person at the same table day after day, each meal is unique. By allowing yourself to surrender to the uniqueness of each meal and each mindful moment, you give in to God and open up, ever so gently, to faith.

Such is the unseen power of prayer, or intention in the name of God.

There are numerous benefits gained by the inner meal practice of surrendering. It opens us up to new and wonderful, even mysterious, possibilities. It reduces feelings of defeat and fear of losing when things don't go exactly our way. It strengthens our faith in all the things we do. It gives us the energy and willingness necessary to take on new challenges and adventures. It centers us on serving others.

Part Two

OUR MINDFUL SEASONINGS

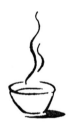

8 – Sacred Listening

There is nothing I can give you
which you do have not;
But there is much, very much, that
while I cannot give it, you can take.

No heaven can come to us unless our
hearts find rest in today. Take heaven!
No peace lies in the future which is not
hidden in this present instant.
Take peace!

The gloom of the world is but a shadow.
Behind it, yet within reach, is joy.
There is a radiance and glory in the
darkness, could we but see, and to see,
we have only to look. I beseech you
to look.

—Fra Giovanni, "A Grateful Heart" (A.D. 1513)

The sacred circle of the family meal is under attack. Since the advent of the TV dinner, the circle has turned outward, with the television at the head of the table. As working parents stay at the workplace longer, the sacred circle atrophies further. Parents desperately want to bring their family together. Yet they compete with the seemingly irresistible pull of television, the Internet, video games, and whatever else happens to be the distraction du jour. The solution is not simply getting the family to convene around the dinner table. That's a start, but it may not produce results if the family is already broken.

I remember the time that a friend of mine told me that he was traveling home for the Christmas holidays. It was the only time during the year that his whole family—his brother, sister, and parents—would be together.

"What do you talk about at your Christmas dinner?" I asked.

"Nothing," he answered plaintively, explaining that other than asking for the mashed potatoes or commenting on the food, his family virtually never spoke at mealtime. This may not seem too bad an alternative for those families where the dinner table turns into a battlefield. Still, a family that says nothing misses the potential to make the family whole and invigorated by seasoning mealtime with vital emotions and meaning. It's somewhat like trying to eat a frozen meal—tasteless, unpleasant, and unsatisfying. This is not to say that food prepared with love and care isn't important. It is. But there is so much more to preparing and enjoying a "centered" family inner meal that stays with you a very, very long time. At its best, the family meal provides many opportunities for learning what matters most—that goes for both parents and children.

Family meals are meant to be integrative and nourishing to us—physically, emotionally, and spiritually. When the family meal turns in this direction, magic happens. This magic cannot happen until we *hear one another.* To truly listen to another is a main course of the family's inner meal. To listen to another is to surrender ourselves, our desires, our impulses. It is to sit back and witness other family members, to give them a moment in the sun, to give them a voice and let them be heard.

Conversely, when we are witnessed by others, we are validated, and our stories gain meaning. The more others listen, the more willing we are to share deeper parts of ourselves. The more the entire story of the family gets revealed, the more we feel the continuity of which we are a vital part. Of course, to hear one another, the family must first be present at the table, not sitting in front of the television or engaged in other activities. But that's just the physical part of the equation. The real question is, How do we listen? One answer is through the ancient, mindful prayer practice of Lectio Divina.

If at first this seems unusual, that's because for many, prayer is solitary and secret, like a birthday wish. But prayer also finds expression communally, as a shared touchstone for family and community to find the sacred within themselves and others. The Jewish Passover seder, a meal of remembrance described earlier, allows young family members to ask questions that are included in the seder prayer book. One of the first questions is "Why is this day different from all the rest?" In this way, all are encouraged to participate and listen. Thus begins the unfolding of this pivotal Jewish story about escape from slavery and the meaning of freedom. This form of communal prayer, with its mixture of reading and listening, creates a deep communication and experience about a shared story. We can use these same methods to season the family meal—or any meal for that matter, because all meals, even those eaten alone, bring us into the human family through which food gains its meaning.

Understanding Lectio Divina

Lectio Divina offers a way to incorporate personal and communal prayer during meals that is easily adapted for use today. Literally translated, *Lectio Divina* means "divine reading," or "sacred reading." But in truth, it's a special form of divine *listening*. It's this listening aspect that sets it apart from other forms of prayer and makes it a uniquely moving practice. What matters, however, is its potential to heal old wounds, strengthen family bonds, and open up channels of communication.

The roots of sacred reading trace back to the desert monks who used it in the second and third centuries. It was also recommended by

Saint Benedict, an Italian monk who was instrumental in developing guidelines for communities of monks—still in use today—for living a life of stability, discipline, and security from which one can find God. His *Rule of Saint Benedict* states: "Reading will always accompany the meals of the brothers." Traditionally, monks practice Lectio Divina, or simply Lectio, at mealtimes, and also at other times during the day.

The practice of Lectio once thrived among early Christians until the late sixteenth century, when it was discouraged for any persons other than monastics. The reason, writes Thelma Hall in *Too Deep for Words*, is that "eventually, it came to be generally accepted that contemplation was an extraordinary grace, restricted to an elite few. This was in total contradiction to the traditional teaching of the first fifteen centuries that contemplation is open to all Christians as the normal development of an authentic spiritual life." Fortunately, Lectio is being rediscovered and is now available to all of us.

Because Lectio may not feel or seem like the prayer we grew up with, it's helpful to first explore the idea of prayer. There exist many kinds of prayer. Among these are centering prayers, mystical prayers, petitionary prayers, loving-kindness prayers, sacramental prayers, protective prayers, prayers for hungry ghosts, prayers for the dying, prayers of abstinence, prayers of forgiveness, and prayers of sacred reading—to name just a few. All, whatever their purpose, have one thing in common: the Word and the Spirit.

Martin Buber, in *I and Thou*, describes the nature of this word-spirit, the same as found within any prayer:

> *Man speaks in many tongues—tongues of language, of art, of action—but the spirit is one; it is response to the You that appears from the mystery. Spirit is word.*

If "Spirit is word," then the Word is Spirit. In the Bible, for instance, the Word of God is inseparable from His action and spirit. One begets the other: "And God said, 'Let there by light'; and there was light...And God said, 'Let there be a firmament in the midst of the waters'...And it was so." Much of the Qur'an's power stems from the fact that it is experienced through Word. Jews read the Word of Torah aloud in temples around the world. Tibetan monks chant mantras—combinations of words and sounds that express holy formulas—which are designed to channel their physical energies into the spiritual realm.

The Word and the Spirit, as practiced in Lectio Divina, still reverberate in Benedictine and Trappist monasteries to this day. Those who use it discover a wonderfully simple and spontaneous way to surrender to deeper meaning. Or they just learn how to listen. The more we surrender, the more we listen; and the more we listen, the more we heal. Not to listen is to shut oneself off from the deeply mending and restorative song of the inner self. Once we surrender to our own song, we can surrender to the song of others.

The more than twenty-five-hundred-year-old *Tao Tê Ching* addresses this in a mystical and eloquent way:

> *If you want to become full,*
> *let yourself be empty.*
> *If you want to be reborn,*
> *let yourself die.*

—Lao-tzu, *Tao Tê Ching* (translated by Stephen Mitchell)

Our Shared Story

Again I have driven up the coast to visit the Mount Calvary Monastery. At 9 A.M. I take a seat in the library, joining twenty-five others who have come to learn the art of holy listening from Brother Timothy Jolley, O.H.C. We form a circle around a massive black wrought-iron fixture with seven lamps that hangs from the center of the high-beamed ceiling. Soft, mottled morning light filters through a shady courtyard into the room. A painting on the wall portrays winged beings in helmets that oddly make them look more like Roman centurions than angels floating above the clouds. Brother Timothy, dressed in his white monk's robe, enters and takes a seat. He starts by talking about the background of Lectio, but returns to what will become a constant theme—the telling and hearing of a story.

This is not just any story. It's *our* story, he tells us. It's how we define who we are, how we identify with our myths, how we connect to our rituals and ceremonies, and ultimately, it's how we *feel* our connection to everybody and everything else around us—from family to friends—deep down in our gut. He then poses a question: What happens when we're cut off and uprooted from our shared stories? One example of this, he says, is the present day cerebral approach to scripture that he believes keeps us separated from ourselves and our community. Lectio simply provides access to those deeper levels of spirituality through our story. We feel its dynamic presence each time our family gathers at the dinner table.

As Brother Timothy speaks, I am reminded of the different paths that yoga provides for Hindus. The intellectual path, *jñana yoga,* is like the cerebral path he's talking about. Lectio, it seems, is probably more like *bhakti yoga*—the path of love, or devotion. But returning to his question, there seems a clear answer. To forget or ignore our story is to lose a part of ourselves or, at the very least, a part of our collective selves. Lectio provides us with the tools to rediscover our shared stories and heritage, both as a family and as a community. And what better place to make that discovery than around the sacred circle of family?

Through Lectio, says Brother Timothy, "the Word becomes incarnate." This makes the process a Eucharistic one, because Lectio nourishes us with the Word and the story of who we are as experienced through God. As you begin to practice Lectio, remember that you don't have to be Christian for it to work and for you to feel the deeper meaning of words. Divine reading is for everyone to learn from and to share communally. Through Lectio, the invisible becomes visible. The experience is something received rather than taken.

Soon the time arrives for our own experience of Lectio, and Brother Timothy instructs each of us to seek out a quiet place on the monastery grounds. Moments later I sit facing a serene garden at the back of Mount Calvary. Yuccas, palms, cactus, spindly aloes, thick bushy jades, and a century plant form a lush and diverse desert landscape. A large bell, sun-blistered red with rust, stands sentinel above the plants. A few feet past the garden, narrow steps lead down to the monastic cells.

In my lap I hold Psalm 84. After a moment of centering, I begin to read, softly. Listening to the words, to my own voice as it comes back to me, startles me at first. Usually, we read for others and are more concerned with the projection, tone, and sound of our voice. But here, in Lectio, my voice is slightly muted, feeling somehow softened and smaller. It's as if my ego has temporarily vacated and made room for the sounds and the listening. The faraway voice and words sound foreign, yet somehow familiar. I imagine that these are words I could have written. My initial read-throughs get me familiar with the entire psalm. There is nothing in it, at first glance, that gives me pause.

Then it happens. There is something about a section that I can't put my finger on. Yet it strikes me. I stop and read:

Those who go through the desolate valley
will find it a place of springs,
for the early rains have covered it
with pools of water.

I read the passage repeatedly, opening myself to its inner meaning. I swallow hard, trying not to analyze. But this verse is obviously mine, intended just for me. As I continue reading, the low, melodious vibration of my voice begins to shake me. Like a mantra it speaks to me of God's presence in the form of hope— hope that exists in "a place of springs," even in the face of my inner doubts and trials. Tears run down my face, and through the blur I continue listening to the words. I realize that the vital spiritual nourishment—"the early rains"—that I need to embark on my inner journey are already provided for me. And the knowing presence that I sense around me now lets me know that these "rains" will prepare me for its successful completion. That my "desolate valley" really contains springs of hope speaks to me deeply. Not only am I moved, but

I feel compassion for all who have journeyed their own desolate valley. I know not why, or how, but God has spoken to me of my story.

I glance at my watch. Forty minutes have passed. Can that be? From the monastery kitchen a monk sings a hymn that breaks the stillness. I do not recognize the hymn, but I do know what it means to sing a song from the heart. All of us, I believe, should dwell in a place where our souls are free to sing, and it saddens me to think that many of us do not. I sit for a moment to watch the stillness and peace of the desert landscape. The deep meaning of the words still echoes throughout me, and I know they will be with me for a long time.

Back in the library after the Eucharist and lunch, we share our Lectio experiences. I feel an immediate kinship with anyone who was touched by the same section of Psalm 84. A few didn't get any clear message, but most "heard" something meant just for them. Each of us is different, and through Lectio we find out more about who we really are. To help us explore our Lectio experience further, Brother Timothy asks us to reflect: What is it about what we have heard or felt that touches us deeply? Because of our encounter, how have we changed? What did we discover about ourselves through Lectio that we didn't know before? After some thought, I realize that Lectio has connected me to my inner self and reestablished my sense of harmony, balance, and wholeness.

Brother Timothy describes how the Navajo Indians use their ceremonies, dances, and paintings to heal and create this same sense of harmony. Since these ceremonies are group events, we spend the afternoon exploring our encounter with God in the context of community. Three people volunteer to read a short passage from the Bible. The first person reads the entire passage, and we sit quietly, reflecting on the words. After a short time, each of us says aloud the particular word or phrase that touches us the most. I am amazed at the diversity of responses.

The passage is read a second time. After another reflective pause, we respond to the feelings that we get from our chosen word or phrase. This we express by saying, "I see..." or "I hear..."

And it brings us all—individually and as a group—to a deeper sense of meaning inherent in our encounter.

The third and final reading leads us into stating what God's word intends for us to change or do. We begin our statements with the words, "I believe God wants me to..." There is no judgment and no rejection. There is only listening and acceptance and acknowledgment.

When we are finished, I am awestruck at the feeling of reverence and quiet that pervades the room. It suddenly dawns on me that I have just witnessed our story. As we do so, the gentle and compassionate presence of God rests among us, in our very midst. This is, then, the first step toward developing a community centered on God. Or a centered family. It is by listening to the words of others, not by drowning them out, that our shared words are given a voice.

Lectio for the Family

The Lectio exercises at the end of this chapter can be hard to grasp if introduced in the family setting without proper preparation and understanding. Whoever introduces Lectio should first practice it alone. You'll have to be the judge about whether your family is ready for Lectio. Active and mindful listening, which Lectio teaches, will help your family learn trust and togetherness.

Begin with baby steps—by using these newly honed listening skills to get your family talking about things that matter: daily frustrations, dreams, successes, hopes, and day-to-day details of life. Next, try introducing a blessing or prayer before dinner. Last, "graduate" to reading small passages from different books, thus teaching the concepts of Lectio without including the direct spiritual elements. Some families may need to experience trust and listening before attempting Lectio as a group. Others may dive in without hesitation. Either way, have patience and compassion with your family. Rediscovering your shared story takes time.

The mindful practice of Lectio exists in many variations. Reading from or discussing the Torah during meals is a Jewish tradition.

The monks of Paramahansa Yogananda's Self-Realization Fellowship, for example, read from the *Spiritual Diary*, which contains
short selections from Yogananda and other sages for every day of
the year. Each day, while eating, they reflect silently on a different
passage. Here's one from a section appropriately called "Practicing
the Presence of God":

> *Once when I was meditating I heard His voice,*
> *whispering: "Thou dost say I am away,* but thou didst
> not come in. *That is why thou dost say I am away. I am*
> *always in. Come in and thou wilst see Me. I am always*
> *here, ready to greet thee."*
> —Paramahansa Yogananda, "Man's Eternal Quest"

Don't wait until tomorrow to put your mindful practices to
work. Strengthen your family's sacred circle beginning today. Be
creative with your selection of readings. Above all, let everyone
have a voice, and you'll open up your own family to a new range of
richly shared experiences—in relation to each other, and in relation
to food.

PRACTICE: LECTIO DIVINA

*This exercise can be used two ways. (1) alone, for indi-
viduals who want to practice Lectio by themselves; and (2) in
family settings at mealtime, when one person "reads" for the others.*

*Lectio Divina is practiced by reading sacred scripture
out loud. But the point is not so much to read as it is to listen to
what you're reading or what is being read. The method is
straightforward. If you're practicing Lectio alone, simply find a
short passage of text—probably no more than a page long—
that you value highly. This sacred writing can be a parable,
fable, blessing, poem, or a psalm.*

Sit comfortably in a chair, but with your back erect. If you meditate, feel free to sit in the lotus position. In either case, hold the passage of sacred text in your lap. Sit silently for a moment and allow yourself to focus your attention.

Begin by setting your intention for the Lectio. This intention could be to hear the word of God, to hear your family's story, or to hear the story that is in your own heart. This is a sacred moment, so if you are practicing alone you should find a place where you will be undisturbed.

Begin reading the passage softly and slowly, from beginning to end. If you want, you can begin by saying, "I hear God saying to me these words." In doing so, we surrender ourselves to divine listening. In the past when the monks of Saint Benedict practiced Lectio, they probably did so in a communal setting, speaking the words softly.

Read the complete passage, allowing yourself to listen to the full meaning of the words. Continue going over the passage, reading it slowly until you feel or sense yourself being drawn to a particular word, phrase, or sentence.

Once you've identified a section of the passage that calls to you, become aware that this might be where God wants you to feel his presence. Now you must open, passively, to receiving God's Word and Spirit as you narrow your reading down to that particular word, phrase, or section. Read this section over and over, allowing its meaning to blossom and come into being for you.

Stay with the reading as long as it takes for you to listen to its meaning as expressed by God. Keep in mind that there is no goal in this exercise. You cannot force God's presence to be revealed. All you can do is make yourself available to hear your Story and sense the deeper meaning of your life today.

Whatever you feel at this moment—sadness, anger, bliss, or happiness—is a valid experience and encounter with God. Even if you become upset, do not try to deny or analyze your feeling. Maybe you feel bored. Maybe you feel frustrated. If so, just ask yourself why. Then gently return to your reading and continue with the section you have chosen.

You may, for example, choose to read the same passage more than once. If so, try not to have any preconceived ideas as to what you will experience. Each reading is unique, and new meanings may reveal themselves to you.

Lectio can be used at mealtime—by reading either for oneself or for others. If one person reads for others, then the listeners simply reflect on the phrase that strikes them. They can reflect silently during the meal, or share their feelings.

There are many benefits gained, both individually and as a group, by the practice of sacred listening. It gives us insights into our deeper purpose. It gives us a sense of inner peace and harmony. It lets us sense God within and around us. It helps us gain empathy for others. It lets us understand the concerns and viewpoints of those in our family. It helps us strengthen the bond between our sacred circle of family and friends. It lets us practice surrendering. It gives others around us a voice and lets us experience the art of listening.

MAKE A LECTIO DIVINA JOURNAL

Keep a journal of your experiences with Lectio. Take care that you do not take notes during the Lectio experience. But if you want to chronicle your experience, do so immediately after your reading. Then again, it's the experience that counts, so don't feel compelled to write anything down.

9 – Ritual Blessings and Chicken Soup

*The ruler of a certain state asked
Confucius about government.
Confucius replied, "Have leaders be leaders,
have administrators be administrators,
have fathers be fathers,
have sons be sons."*

*The ruler said, "Good! Of a truth,
if leaders do not lead,
administrators do not administer,
fathers do not behave as fathers,
and sons do not behave as sons,
then even if there were grain,
how could I eat of it?"*

—Confucius, from "The Essential Confucius"
(translated by Thomas Cleary)

It is a sunny, but cool day as I leave the cottage and get in my car. Four monks climb in for the ride to a nearby restaurant. By providing food to the monks, I take part in an ancient ritual offering and custom that has existed for almost three thousand years.

When I ask where they would like to go, they recommend a buffet-style, Chinese restaurant by the name of Paradise. I smile to myself, wondering if it's the food or the name that they like best. Since Burmese Buddhist monks do not eat after noontime, we arrive at 11 A.M., when the restaurant opens. Monks usually eat together, separate from the laity. But one of them pulls out a chair and I sit with them.

We eat slowly and quietly, though there is much attentiveness to everyone's needs—such as filling teacups and sharing food. There is even some spontaneous laughter as occurs at any meal where friends gather. The food is excellent, and the wide selection gives all of us the opportunity to eat a balanced diet. Near the end of the meal, one of the monks brings a plateful of orange slices for all to share. Finally, we're done and it's not yet 11:45.

Before we rise from the table, the monks become quiet, their concentration apparent. They chant, in ancient Pali, a ritual prayer from what are known as the Protective Suttas—to bless the welfare of humankind. The focused vibration of their voices produces a small ripple of centering and soothing energy that spreads throughout the restaurant.

> *May all dangers be erased.*
> *May worry and illness vanish.*
> *May you never have any misfortunes.*
> *May you have joy and long life.*
>
> *Those who are gifted with the*
> *nature of piety and who always revere*
> *the elders, these four gifts shall*
> *prosper:—namely longevity, beauty,*
> *happiness and strength.*

Sacred Meaning for Daily Life and Community

Probably since the beginning of human tribal societies, rituals have played a role in how we adapt to change, act in a given situation, and relate to the world around us. At the tribal level, ritual offers meaning by reaffirming the divine order through some physical manifestation or expression—such as a ceremonial dance or a chant. At a more fundamental level, it forms the invisible glue that holds everything together. It makes new and even uneasy social situations easier to handle—from shaking hands and greeting strangers to waiting in line at the market. It offers a set of unwritten rules that guide us through daily life and help us reach our human potential.

An average meal contains a certain amount of unspoken ritual. It can be subtle, like the way that we wait until everyone is served before eating. Or it can be conspicuous, like recitation of grace before a meal. Sacred ritual adds meaning to meals, which is why it's a vital inner meal practice. Ritual may seem trivial, but historically, ritual meals were even worth dying for. In *The Jewish Dietary Laws*, Rabbi Samuel H. Dresner writes that "the aged scribe Eleazar submitted to death rather than permit pig's flesh to pass his lips and is one of the first recorded martyrs of Israel."

Mindful and sacred rituals give expression to our beliefs and provide us with comfort and hope. This is why, in times of hardship, rituals are what we hold on to most tightly. They bind us to the warmth and comfort of the familiar. The recipes of the women incarcerated in the Nazi death camp Theresienstadt, as collected in the book *In Memory's Kitchen*, are a testament to the comforting and sustaining power of ritual:

> *Two sisters by the door, a pair*
> *Their harmony is something rare*
> *A love of cooking both do share*
> *But it's platonic, their cupboard is bare*
> *The food they had brought no longer there.*

—Wilhelmina (Mina) Pächter

Many Chinese, for example, provide ritual offerings of food to a kitchen god who they believe watches the family during the year. They do this to thank the kitchen god for the year's bounty of food. From this offering springs the hope that the kitchen god will recommend their household to the more supreme Jade Emperor who resides among the heavens. In Hong Kong, families often place salted fish at the altar of the kitchen god. In China, starchy and sticky sweet cakes are offered. If the Jade Emperor is pleased with the kitchen god's report, then the family is rewarded in the coming year with prosperity and plentiful food for their cupboards.

The thoughts of Confucius on the topic of ritual are worth considering. He lived at a time, in the sixth century B.C., when a once powerful dynasty was no longer able to maintain a unifying peace. Basically, he saw tradition and ritual as spreading order, peace, and security among our community and society. He believed that tradition best served society when it was deliberately created and sustained through effort and intelligence. Confucius's concept of *li*—sacred ritual or ceremony—is tied to how well a ritual serves society. Our dignity as humans depends on the ceremony, especially when we attach it to our community and our family.

There is a story in the *Analects*—a collection of Confucius's sayings—where one of his disciples asks about children's responsibility to their parents and whether it is good enough to simply take care of a parent's physical needs. Confucius responds that even "dogs and horses" get fed. This story illustrates that the caring, respect, and devotion associated with the act of giving food are what matter most of all.

According to the teachings of Confucius, it is our human calling—if not a solemn human duty—to transform the act of obtaining nourishment into a ceremony of special significance. *Li* helps us discover our true dignity and grace. Ceremony is, after all, what separates us from other animals. We enable the sacred to exist by using ritual to serve and ennoble others. When we serve others, ritual becomes communal, and it is here that we transcend the ego to become part of the holy community.

Ritual and Mindful Meals of Remembrance

Outside my cottage windows a palm-sized bird flutters its wings rapidly, its soft white underside exposed in flight. It zips from tree to grass and back to tree, looking for food. On the ground, it hops two or three times, bobs its tail, then it's airborne, alternately flapping and gliding through the air in what seems a never-ending movement. It repeats this series of actions over and over, again and again. There is comfort, I muse, in knowing what will come next, even when we really don't.

I watch the little bird for a short while, then walk over to the monastery. I see that a family has come to offer food for the monks—a Theravadan Buddhist tradition. After the monks finish eating, the family heats up more food and settles in the monastery dining room to enjoy their own lunch. When they find out I am staying here, they kindly invite me to join them. I sit next to Kenny, a well-spoken man who strikes up a conversation during the meal.

"Are you meditating?" he asks me.

"Yes," I answer, "and writing a book about the spiritual aspects of food."

I mention a few of the Buddha's ideas, and he turns strangely silent. I notice his solemnness, but say nothing.

Soon, the discussion turns into a lively debate about which restaurants and markets have the best food. Two young brothers scamper around the table offering their relatives paper cups filled with water. The boys become the topic of conversation, with everybody wondering why they are so hyperactive. The adults seem to agree that sugar-based sodas are the culprit. We sit and talk a while longer. After the dishes are washed, everyone moves outside, ready to go.

Kenny looks at me, deep in thought. "Today is our Day of Remembrance, to honor and remember our ancestors," he says solemnly. I nod back, now understanding his earlier silence. While I knew that many traditions had ritual meals for this kind of thing, I didn't have the faintest idea I had just eaten at one.

Everyone grows quiet as Kenny tells me that his sister died

this past year, of cancer. This is a moment of acknowledgment and courage, his way of making greater peace with his loss. His family, it turns out, had planned to honor her memory on this special Chinese Remembrance Day, or All Soul's Day. Before the meal, as part of a ritual offering, he and his family had prayed and placed food by the statue of Buddha in the monastery. The topic of conversation eventually shifts, and we've made it through an uneasy moment. We all smile again, and the family says good-bye to me and one of the monks.

This remembrance through the ritual of a family meal is also a part of other wisdom traditions. Jewish tradition, for example, calls this a "meal of recovery," and it is contributed to by the family and friends of those who are grieving. Food is brought to the home of the mourners in baskets. In this way, mourners are saved having to prepare their own meals during the first difficult days of their loss. This is considered an important act of loving-kindness, or mitzvah. Ritual meals like this one—also practiced by Muslims and others—let us know that life goes on. We can honor and hallow the past even as we acknowledge and serve the needs of the present.

A Model Ritual Meal

The Jewish Sabbath, or Shabbat, illustrates how to transform the dinner table into a sacred altar. But it is the ability of this ritual meal to successfully combine several ritual elements that makes it a model for other Jewish holidays. Ostensibly, *Shabbat* in Hebrew means "rest," but this is the kind of rest that allows time to develop and spiritually replenish one's soul.

Even the person-to-person greeting is ritualized on this day with the words *Shabbat Shalom*: "May you have a peaceful Sabbath." In all, the Sabbath reminds Jews that God created the world and lets them reflect on their freedom. It also connects them with the natural world and with others who celebrate Sabbath.

The rituals used for Sabbath include the presence of candles, wine, and bread, and the creation of an environment of beauty, harmony, and peace. Thus, the presentation of the dinnerware, table setting, and food for this sacred meal is as attractive and elegant as possible. Instead of plain bread, for example, beautifully braided challah is used. The participants also dress in their best clothes.

The reason for this beautification—indeed, the reason for Sabbath—is to help us mind-shift away from our daily routines and mundane struggles. In the process, we shift into a sublime and spiritual place. It is considered a sin, for example, to worry about the past or be sad during the Sabbath. The whole point is to cleanse our souls, be joyful in the moment, and be at peace with ourselves, others, and nature.

Shabbat starts with a prayer over the lighting of candles at sundown:

> *Blessed are You, Lord our God, Eternal One, Who allows us to bring the peace of Shabbat into our homes by kindling these lights.*

This symbolically brings light and truth into the home. It also makes a break from the workweek that has come before. Blessings for the wine and bread—described in chapter 5—follow next. Customarily, the specially braided bread, or challah, is covered with a decorated cloth until the prayer for the wine is said. As tradition has it, this saves the challah from the embarrassment of having the wine blessed first!

These blessings for the wine and challah hallow the food and the creation of the world. The Sabbath meal itself is cooked prior to sundown. Some believe that the proper choice of food, such as the traditional chicken soup, also plays a part in sanctifying the Sabbath.

After sundown—when the Sabbath's injunction against work begins—food may be warmed, but not cooked. In fact, the use of electricity and other mechanical devices during the Sabbath is forbidden. This is a time to walk, to slow down, and to feel our sacred place in nature. This is also a time to celebrate by singing traditional Hebrew songs.

A *Shabbat Song*, as written in the *Siddur Sim Shalom* prayer book, encourages participants to sing these words:

The sun on the treetops no longer is seen.
Come, let us welcome Shabbat, the true Queen.
Behold her descending, the holy, the blessed,
and with her God's angels of peace and of rest.
Come now, come now, our Queen, our Bride.

Sabbath concludes with the making of *havdalah,* a ritual that acknowledges the end of the Sabbath spirit. Short prayers are either sung or recited while sipping wine, lighting a candle, and inhaling sweet spices. Traditionally, the sweet smell of nutmeg and other spices symbolizes optimism for the coming week. These actions are meant to provide comfort and solace for the loss of sacred time and the return to secular life.

By making a separation between the secular and sacred, Sabbath encourages the weekly practice of a spiritual approach to living. Abraham Heschel, in his book *The Sabbath,* explains that instead of trying to dominate the world as we do six days out of the week, on the Sabbath we have as our purpose to "try to dominate the self." The real power and meaning of Sabbath's ritual observances, says Heschel, come from a shift in our perspective. The Sabbath day is unlike any other because it sanctifies and hallows the world of time:

> *The meaning of the Sabbath is to celebrate time rather*
> *than space. Six days a week we live under the tyranny*
> *of things of space; on the Sabbath we try to become at-*
> *tuned to **holiness in time**. It is a day on which we are*
> *called upon to share in what is eternal in time, to turn*
> *from the results of creation to the mystery of creation;*
> *from the world of creation to the creation of the world.*

Sacred rites, however, reveal their spiritual quality only when their deepest meanings and metaphors are known. Simply to wash our hands before a meal or to beat on a sacred drum without knowledge of the wellspring from which the ritual flows is to restrict its spiritual power and keep it inert. When ritually washing hands, for example, water becomes inseparable from the blessing that accompanies it. It becomes a holy medium—a spiritual spring that cleanses and purifies the soul as much as it washes the hands.

Some rites, such as those of the Native American Sioux Indians, employ sacred objects like the pipe and the drum to sanctify their rituals. For Black Elk, the Native American Sioux holy man, sacred objects are holy vessels because of the meaning they hold:

> *Since the drum is often the only instrument used in our sacred rites, I should perhaps tell you here why it is especially sacred and important to us. It is because the round form of the drum represents the whole universe, and its steady strong beat is the pulse, the heart, the throbbing at the center of the universe. It is as the voice of **Wakan-Tanka**, and this sound stirs us and helps us to understand the mystery and power of all things.*

—"The Sayings of Black Elk," in *The World's Religions*

Bringing Ritual Prayer Home

We live in a world that seems to grow more secularized day by day. While many of us search for meaning, we may not realize that ritual is the perfect spiritual appetizer. Not only that, it's a relatively simple element to add to our personal and family life. When an entire culture, religion, or family shares in ritual, its members experience a deep feeling of order and meaning.

It's natural for us to practice a ritual we're already familiar with. But what if we don't have an established ritual of our own? Trying on someone else's ritual can be like trying on a new pair of gloves or shoes: we need to wear them for a while until they grow comfortable. Rituals are like that.

I can remember when I first went to the Eucharist with a Catholic friend out of curiosity. I was only a teenager at the time, and I did not feel comfortable enough to take communion, let alone bow my head. I felt as if I had entered a foreign country—and the Latin spoken in services at that time didn't help. Later, while in college, I went to communion with a classmate and experienced it for the first time—this time out of courtesy. It was not until recently that I had the opportunity to experience the Eucharist again. This time, however, I was able to more honestly experience it through my communion with others and a deeper understanding of its ultimate meaning. Thus, out of a deep sense of respect I was able to feel it filtered through my own set of beliefs.

Nowadays, whether I am alone or with others, I like to say a silent blessing of thanks and loving-kindness before my meal. When my immediate family gathers for holidays or a family reunion, I'll say a few words of thanks to God for bringing us together. But I couldn't imagine trying to say even the most innocuous prayer or blessing at a table where it wasn't welcomed and agreed upon. As much as we may want to bring the sacred into our lives, we need to respect others.

Given that you want to develop a mindful mealtime tradition for your family or yourself, the world is open to you with a cornucopia of blessings and other rituals. All that you need to do is set the precedent by making ritual part of your daily tradition. By doing so you show your gratefulness for the blessing of life that food provides you. You acknowledge that the smallest morsel of food is a miracle to be hallowed. Do so proudly, and with dignity—wherever you happen to be.

PRACTICE: FINDING YOUR RITUAL BLESSING

If you want to find a before- or after-mealtime blessing for a particular wisdom tradition, you have many books and resources from which to choose. For example, A Grateful Heart *contains 365 blessings that are categorized according to the seasons. Marianne Williamson's* Illuminata *offers a call to love through prayers of all kinds and for all occasions. Daily Readings from* Prayer and Praises in the Celtic Tradition *is an anthology alive with Celtic spiritual insight.*

Any journey takes a certain amount of planning, patience, and practice. So whatever blessing you choose to use, practice it repeatedly. This gives meaning to a ritual. It soon becomes an established tradition that you and your family can cherish.

Anything that you decide to recite and make sacred becomes so. You might want to find a prayer that blesses the food, acknowledges God, emphasizes the togetherness of your family, or recognizes any number of things. It can even be a moment of silence given as thanks. Try to learn the roots, the history, and the tradition behind the writings you take as your own. When you recite a prayer, you are invoking Word and Spirit as old as human language itself.

Once you find a blessing that feels right, try making it part of your daily life. Wisdom traditions tend to use the same blessings over and over. The repetition creates a sense of shared experience that comes from knowing that your prayer or blessing is being used by countless others.

There are many benefits to finding and practicing your own inner meal ritual blessing. It helps make an important, everyday part of life sacred. It unites the family through a moment of centering. It establishes a family or personal tradition. It offers strength, faith, and comfort. It encourages a sense of well-being that comes from keeping a commitment. It helps develop and enrich the connection to a particular faith. It brings a sense of consistency, serenity, and peace to daily life.

10 – Giving and Receiving a Cup of Tea

With a bowl of tea, peace can truly spread.

—Soshitsu Sen XV, "Tea Life, Tea Mind"

Through the cottage windows the sky has darkened. I walk over to the main building as raindrops pelt the ground. I was gone for the day to attend to business and want to tell the monks I am back. When I step outside again the rain has stopped. I walk the grounds, wondering what unseen hand orchestrates an entire landscape. The grass, the trees—everything takes on a richer, deeper shade of color. The clouds reflect an uncanny hue of blue. Small brown birds swoop between branches, singing. A large black crow sits regally on a telephone pole stretching its wings. Everything moves, alive and emboldened by the rain. Leaves on every tree flutter in the breeze. Fresh puddles of rainwater shimmer.

I crane my neck to look up at a large pine tree, then over to the little yellow cottage where I write. It seems fragile in comparison. Its thin clapboard walls and scalloped white molding have shielded me from the outside world and its distractions. I know I will leave here soon, but I want to keep it in my heart, to use it whenever I need to find peace. Suddenly, I feel awed—no, humbled—by everything around me. I think for a moment how the monks have shown me loving-kindness and compassion during my stay. They have shared their food, provided me with shelter, and helped me find that quiet place inside myself so that I might reach my quest. That, too, will remain in my heart.

Offering and receiving. Giving and taking. Serving and accepting. At first glance the poles of these two sets of opposites seem destined never to meet. There is no middle ground, no mutual foundation. The former is tainted with sainthood, the latter with selfhood. These apparently contrary and dissimilar ideas, however, are not meant to be separated from one another. In truth they make a quite elegant fit, together forming the most beautiful mosaic of a complete and full human heart. To experience their true essence is to dissolve our prejudices and preconceptions about what it means to give and to receive.

The Way of Tea

At first glance, the inner meal practice of the Japanese tea ceremony unifies the concepts of offering and receiving. Actually, it does much more than that. The secular tea ceremony derives from an approach to life and a school of thought known as *Chado*, or the Way of Tea. The tea ceremony provides an exquisitely mindful model for bridging the gap that exists in our modern lives between harmony and commotion, thoughtfulness and carelessness, aesthetics and coarseness, respect and selfishness.

Roots of the tea ceremony trace back to twelfth-century China and Zen Buddhism. Traditionally, Chinese monks used tea to increase their awareness and concentration during meditation. Japanese monks who visited China brought tea back with them to Japan. The sect of Buddhism, which Huston Smith calls "the Buddhism that Taoism profoundly influenced, namely *Ch'an* (Zen in Japanese)," asks us to look for the greatest meaning in the smallest of life's events. Zen looks beneath the surface to uncover the oneness and the sublime that exist in the mundane. As inherent in the minimalist Zen phrase "chop wood; carry water," meaning comes not from what we do, but from the way in which we do our daily work.

The flashes of insight that form the essence of Zen abound in many different tales. One well-known story, as told by David Scott and Tony Doubleday in *The Elements of Zen*, describes the encounter between a ninth-century Chinese Zen master Joshu and a visiting monk:

> *A monk once came to Joshu at breakfast time and said:*
> *'I have just entered this monastery. Please teach me.'*
> *'Have you eaten your porridge yet?' asked Joshu.*
> *'Yes, I have,' replied the monk.*
> *'Then you had better wash your bowl,' said Joshu.*

This story makes the point that in Zen, meaning resides in the ordinary. To "wash your bowl" is to do the work from which the essence of all knowing can be discovered. Understanding these origins, it comes as no surprise to us that during a tea ceremony the utensils are cleaned and washed as the ceremony progresses. Even during those ceremonies that include a full meal, guests are expected to clean their plates of all food.

Originally, tea in Japan represented wealth and was enjoyed exclusively by Japanese Zen priests and royalty in the most elegant surroundings and using the most expensive utensils. Over time, the tea ceremony shifted away from pretension. A new, more humble, unassuming, less-is-more ceremony evolved rooted in the essence and aesthetics of Zen.

It wasn't until the sixteenth century and a tea master named Sen Rikyu, however, that the practices and principles of tea developed into the Way of Tea. But since Zen Buddhism absorbed ideas from Taoism, concepts of Tao are also part of the Way of Tea. Legend has it that the tea ceremony began when Lao Tzu—the mystical "Old One" who wrote the twenty-five-hundred-year-old *Tao Tê Ching*, or *Book of the Way and Its Virtue*—was offered a cup of tea by a disciple. It is in this essential Taoist scripture that the oneness of the Way, or reality, and the means of being in harmony with the universe are revealed.

Opening up to the Way of Tea means looking at the kitchen, the meal, the guests, and the hosts in an entirely new way. Here, everything is used in creating a mindful inner meal. Nothing is tossed out; nothing is wasted. These principles form the cornerstone of the Urasenke School of tea—with its more than 2 million followers worldwide. The four basic principles that guide this school's Way of Tea are the values of harmony, purity, respect, and tranquility. Through practicing these principles, we complete what is incomplete—within ourselves and the within the world around us. This means finding peace in our anxiety, confidence in our unease, and harmony in the surrounding chaos.

It is almost magical to think that a single tea ceremony can hold all these energies simultaneously in the same place. Somehow, through the almost alchemical application of diligence, mindful action, and serenity, it succeeds. At the same time, guest and host act as cooperative architects of beauty and perfection.

> *True beauty could be discovered only by one who mentally completed the incomplete. The virility of life and art lay in its possibilities for growth. In the tearoom it is left for each guest in imagination to complete the total effect in relation to himself.*
> —Kakuzo Okakura, *The Book of Tea*

It is a Saturday morning as I drive south from Los Angeles to a tea ceremony class. Tomiko Numano, a tea *sensei*, or master, from the Urasenke School of tea, has invited me to join in. Looking for a school-like structure on the residential street, I wonder if I have made a wrong turn. Again I check the address, and walk up to a single-level home. After ringing the bell, a student leads me to the tea room. It is not located in the backyard as I half expect, but stands in the house, almost like a home within a home.

Although I have arrived on time, the all-morning class is already in progress. I enter through one of the tea room's sliding doors, and I am greeted by Tomiko, who is kneeling and attired in a traditional tea kimono. With an air of elegance and grace she pauses from her class and asks me to sit. I find a comfortable corner—as comfortable as one can be sitting on a tatami mat constructed from rice straw.

Class continues, and I watch, mesmerized. I feel as though I've been transported back centuries in time. Soft light filters gently through the rice-paper-covered sliding doors. A misty hush of steam vents from a black cast-iron teapot. The natural, unvarnished redwood and Douglas fir beams of the tea room add nature's warming touch. Sitting cross-legged, I'm overwhelmed with a feeling of tranquility. The world of commotion and care beyond the tea room fades like an evanescent rainbow.

Tomiko gently corrects each student as they go through what looks like a simple routine but is actually a complex ritual. Learning the tea ceremony can take years of devoted and diligent practice. Each minuscule movement is choreographed, each filled with mindfulness and total attention.

A student slowly, almost painstakingly, lifts a delicate, long-handled wooden scoop filled with *matcha*, green powdered tea leaves, and pours this into a ceramic bowl. Using a *chasen*, a bamboo whisk, she whisks the tea into what looks like a frothy green soup, then carries a bowl of tea over to me. When she bows and offers the bowl, I take it. Although I am unsure of the protocol. Tomiko guides me. She explains that I am to take three sips from the bowl, drinking it all, and then wipe the rim clean with three deliberate swipes from a thin napkin.

The tea is thick and green and pulpy, unlike any I've ever had, yet hearty, satisfying, somehow woody, and quite possibly the best tea I have ever tasted. This, I learn, is *koicha*, a thick tea that is enjoyed during one part of an entire tea ceremony. I nod and return the bowl.

Class pauses for a break. Tomiko invites me to an actual tea ceremony the next week, and I happily accept.

"It is the first tea of the year," she adds.

"First tea?"

"Yes, we celebrate the New Year with tea."

Though I'm excited about experiencing the first major tea event of the year, I have seen enough to know that the tea ceremony is a fully participatory event. Guests play an important and sacred role, and I ask her whether I am prepared for a full-fledged tea ceremony. Tomiko simply smiles and asks me which of the two teas ceremonies I would prefer—the one that will include several Los Angeles tea masters or the one with the students. I want to say "tea masters," but feel more comfortable with the students. It's all set for next Sunday—First Tea with a theme of The Year of the Tiger.

Halfway through the week I get a call from Tomiko. The student tea ceremony is too crowded, she says. Would I mind switching to the other one? "Sure, that's fine," I reply nervously.

As First Tea approaches, I decide to follow the words of sixteenth-century tea master Rikyu regarding being a guest at any dinner:

> *Fight your shame.*
> *Throw out your pride and learn all you can from others.*
> *This is the basis of a successful life.*

On the day of First Tea, a crisp and breezy Sunday, I arrive at tea master Tomiko's house midmorning. I am greeted by Mr. Numano, Tomiko's husband, who is dressed in traditional Japanese attire. With a hearty handshake, he ushers me in to the living room, where all the guests meet one another and get comfortable.

The house, I notice, has been transformed. A large, colorful banner hangs from the perimeter walls. Thin, square cushions rest on all the chairs and sofas. Mr. Numano introduces me to the other guests, all Japanese. I sit next to Sam, an outgoing older gentleman who has built several tea rooms. All the wood must be perfectly cut and notched, especially the room's round support beam, he explains. Harmony with nature means fitting the wood together with no nails. When I express amazement at this, Sam concedes with a conspiratorial wink and smile that his tea room at home may contain one or two nails.

New guests arrive, including a diminutive woman in her eighties who, I learn, is the honored "First Guest" and a highly revered tea master known throughout the United States. The role of First Guest is to ask questions about the history of ancient utensils, ease the flow and tone of conversation, and help create social harmony. We're already at ease when we leave the greeting area for the ceremony to begin. A complete, formal tea ceremony like this one contains several phases, including a thick tea, a thin tea, and a full meal. The whole ceremony takes up to three hours or more.

We first enter a large room arranged like a tea room. Here we are formally introduced to one another and have the opportunity to admire the workmanship of some ancient utensils. A sweet, sticky dessert covered in a red wrapper stimulates our taste buds—or at least it did mine—in preparation for the tea.

As the ceremony continues I discover that the *teishu*, the host or hostess, does not eat, and is only concerned with the aspect of serving. Here I am to experience the first of many lessons about the power of giving and receiving, and the joy that exists when something is given without obligation and received without shame.

We move outside into an immaculately kept garden. Tomiko sprinkles water over the plants and the ground by a bamboo fountain, then glides silently out of the way. Even this *roji*, or dewy garden path, is a formalized part of the ceremony. One by one we step onto stones leading to the fountain. I step, as in a walking meditation up to the fountain, which gurgles like a small stream. I place my hands underneath, allowing the cool waters to purify and cleanse my hands and face before I enter the tea room for thick tea. Once inside,

I follow everyone's movements without a major faux pas.

While water simmers in an antique black kettle that sits down low over a sunken hearth, Tomiko uses an embroidered silk tea cloth to clean the utensils. The tea bowl, the cup-shaped lacquer tea container, the bamboo tea whisk, the slender tea scoop—all these are wiped clean with slow, measured strokes. I watch with rapt attention, realizing that even by cleaning we can create something that is beautiful and beyond words.

Tomiko carefully scoops up a ladleful of hot water from the kettle and pours it into the tea bowl. As she whisks the *matcha* into thick tea, her deliberate, mindful movements establish a sense of calm throughout the tea room. Now it is time to share the tea. The bowl is handed respectfully, with a bow, to the First Guest. Soon, each of us savors our three long sips, wipes clean the rim of the bowl, and passes the tea to the person on our left. We also watch as the nearly two-hundred-year-old handcrafted utensils used to make our thick tea are ritually cleaned and then passed around for our appreciation.

At the front of the tea room, in a small alcove, hangs a handwritten scroll. A Zen saying, perhaps? I decide not to bluntly ask. I enjoy the simple but elegant *chabana*, or flower arrangement, consisting of a strand of straw and two red and white camellias—colors signifying happiness. The spareness of the straw draws my memory back to the sparse Chicago winters of my youth. But what strikes me most? The spontaneous sharing of laughter and purposeful conversation in the midst of focused attention, peace, and serenity. Conversation, like tea, is not done to excess, and not wasted. Harmony within and without.

At the conclusion of thick tea, we move outside once more. We sit on chairs under a loosely woven bamboo covering that shields us from the sun's glare. As we enjoy *usucha*, or thin tea, the group becomes even more energetic and lively. With anticipation, we re-enter the house for the final phase of the tea ceremony—the meal.

I sit cross-legged on a small pillow at one of three long tables. Here, we are treated to a sumptuous meal of sushi, sashimi, miso soup, Japanese vegetables, and hot sake. There is much conversation, laughter, and a continuous offering of food and drink. I learn that proper etiquette dictates eating all the food on the plate. After I have eaten all the rice in my rice bowl, for example, one of the servers fills it with a small portion of water—which I first swirl around to cleanse the bowl, and then drink. Even when eating, the tea ceremony embodies the Zen practice of cleaning as you go.

But it is what happens after the meal that seems to sum up the essence of tea. When we have finished eating I am surprised to learn that our ceremony will conclude with each of us taking part in a lottery to choose gifts provided by our hosts. A tea server holds out a large, black-lacquered bowl containing phrases that match up with gifts. All the phrases relate in some way to the First Tea and Year of the Tiger theme.

I reach in the bowl and pick one. Since all phrases are in Japanese, the friendly guest to my left offers to translate. But when she sees the small inscription, her face turns red and she covers her mouth in mute astonishment.

"What does it say?" I ask, full of curiosity.

"It's from our history, very famous," she says, leaving me hanging a moment longer. "Do you know the words, *tora tora tora?*"

"Yes, I've heard them," I answer vaguely, but the only thing I remember is something about an old World War II movie titled *Tora! Tora! Tora!*

"Code words," she says almost hushed. "These were the code words for 'Attack the United States. Attack the United States.'"

The stunned look on my face lasts only a moment before she unravels the mystery of why this phrase is in the lottery.

"The code words *tora tora tora* really mean 'tiger tiger tiger,' for Year of the Tiger," she says.

At last the moment comes when Tomiko raises a gift and calls out the now infamous words. I wave my inscription in the air. Like a sudden bolt of electricity, the whole room jolts with astonishment. "I was born in the Year of the Tiger," I say, finding this double coincidence even more amusing. The irony of all this jars us into simultaneous laughter and epiphany.

I look at the kind, generous, sincere people before me. They are open enough to invite a stranger into their home and share in a sacred and intimate ceremony and meal. I consider history, and my father—a man who served his country in World War II in the Pacific and who witnessed firsthand the devastation at Hiroshima. There are those in the family who say he was a different man when he returned home to his wife and to a son he had never before met. Together, we bear the scars of our histories, there is no doubt. But together, as moments like mine in the tea room show, we can learn that it is not so easy to consider one an enemy after inviting him or her into your home to share in peace, harmony, and a bowl of tea. It may be near impossible.

I like to think that the lesson of tea's inner meal can be used at any meal and with all guests. For then, we do as Soshitsu Sen XV says:

In my own hands I hold a bowl of tea; I see all of nature represented in its green color. Closing my eyes I find green mountains and pure water within my own heart.
Silently sitting alone and drinking tea, I feel these become part of me. What is the most wonderful thing for people like myself who follow the Way of Tea? My answer: the oneness of host and guest created through 'meeting heart to heart' and sharing a bowl of tea.

PRACTICE: MINDFUL MEAL PREPARATION

Have you ever prepared a meal, cleaned the dishes, or swept the kitchen floor feeling only the drudgery of these acts and wondering why your chores aren't easier? At one time or another we've probably all felt this way. One concept of Zen and the Way of Tea is that of cleaning up as you go. This cleaning applies to your preparation and to your mind. Both, when cleaned constantly, let you live in the moment.

In Zen, the more mundane and difficult the task, the more useful it is considered for spiritual training. Kakuzo Okakura, in the classic The Book of Tea, *writes that "in the caretaking of the monastery...the novices were committed the lighter duties, while to the most respected and advanced monks were given the most irksome and menial tasks. Such services formed a part of the Zen discipline and every least action must be done absolutely perfectly."*

Consider this the next time you are about to chop vegetables or wipe the table clean—for even the most simple actions become sacred when performed with a sense of total commitment and caring. Use this practice whenever you feel distracted or scattered, and need to get centered and calm.

As you begin preparation for your meal, reflect on your intent. Your intent may be to prepare a meal with love, caring, and attention. To waste no food and waste no motion. To clean up while preparing. To remain centered and in the moment during every step of the preparation. To establish a sense of purity through the sacred act of cleaning.

Think about the ways in which you can accomplish some of your objectives. It might help to unclutter your mind—and your kitchen—by rearranging your kitchen utensils or installing that extra shelf. Or to go about collecting all the ingredients and utensils you need for your meal before starting. In this way, you won't need to break your concentration when you suddenly can't find the colander. Also, give yourself enough time. By doing so, you're also recognizing that this meal is special—that it isn't a five-minute microwave affair.

The practice of mindful preparation offers many benefits. It helps one's ability to center and give every task its due. It teaches thankfulness for the opportunity to practice diligence in all work. It reduces mistakes in preparing food. It increases the beauty of meals by increasing greater attention to detail. It fosters teamwork and responsibility.

PRACTICE: TEA CEREMONY

The four ideals of the tea ceremony—purity, harmony, tranquility, and respect—can be experienced on a daily basis through this inner meal practice. If this is a path you choose to cultivate, you may find that it brings a sense of meaning and beauty to all of life's actions.

Purity. The roots of purity are nourished by cleanliness and order. With the tea ceremony, cleanliness begins in each pantry where utensils and foodstuffs are stored, in each kitchen where food is prepared, in each tea room where guests are served, and in each garden where guests purify themselves in cool water. Through our earnest effort of wiping away the grime, removing impurities, and creating a tidy and fastidious environment, we symbolically sweep away the clutter and confusion of the physical world. Use this concept to clean your kitchen, organize your work space, and unclutter your immediate world. Know that in this way you can empty your mind from the details and debris that obscure your true inner self.

Harmony. Any meal can mirror the harmony of the season and environment. Make a point of finding out what foods are seasonal and local. They may be the freshest. Try experimenting with new, seasonal combinations that you haven't tried before. Shop and choose your foods in the market with the same mindful attention that you give to kitchen preparation.

Tranquility. Create tranquility by reflecting on how you can create an island of space and time for your family to share the meal. Turn off your phone during mealtime. Try to get all the family members agree to sacrifice something so as not to let interruptions intrude on this sacred time together.

Respect. Create respect for others at the table by listening to them and letting them have a voice. You can do this by invoking a prayer or sacred reading, or finding another way to involve everyone. Help your family members understand the benefits of making dinner a priority, arriving on time, and participating.

The inner meal practice of emulating the tea ceremony provides several advantages. It creates more wholesome and natural meals. It lets us experience a sense of harmony and peace—within ourselves and in connection to others. It helps bring respect and discipline to the dinner table. It makes every individual important by letting each hold a sacred responsibility.

11 – The Monk's Diet

*If we live in mindfulness, we are no
longer poor, because our practice of
living in the present moment makes us
rich in joy, peace, understanding,
and love.*

—Thich Nhat Hanh, "Our Appointment
with Life"

Why does anyone become a monk or a nun? Why do men and
women willingly leave the world of affairs behind them? Why do
they seek solitude and communities of others who are like-minded?
Plato and others extolled the benefits of wisdom to be gained by
escaping or withdrawing from the world for periods of time. In
Brother Juniper's Bread Book, Brother Peter Reinhart writes that
"spiritual discipline and practice, *ascesis* in Greek, is for the purpose of conquering the passions." To pursue our human perfection in these ways is to realize the potential for spiritual awakening, and in particular, to harvest the rich and fertile ground that
comes naturally through certain food practices.

One thing common to monks—be they Benedictine, Trappist, Buddhist, or Hindu—is the use of food to encounter spiritual union and to liberate consciousness from hunger, desire, pain, and ignorance. Food is neither indulged in nor used to satisfy emotional desires and attachments. Rather, it acts as sustenance for maintaining physical health and conscious awareness. Saint Benedict stresses in his *Rule* that "above all overindulgence is avoided, lest a monk experience indigestion. For nothing is so inconsistent with the life of any Christian as overindulgence. Our Lord says: *Take care that your hearts are not weighed down with overindulgence* (Luke 21:34)."

Every living thing is maintained by food, and in some wisdom traditions the nutrients in food are thought to contribute to an increase in spiritual capacity. Many monks are vegetarian, though not all. Hindu and Taoist monks, for example, follow an exclusively vegetarian diet. Certain sects of Buddhist monks, such as Tibetans and Mahayanists, observe vegetarianism, while the Theravadans do not. Traditionally, monks following the *Rule of Saint Benedict* were vegetarians, though that is now often voluntary. This is not to say that vegetarianism has the market on spirituality. For monks, it's just as important how they eat as *what* they eat. Each monastic community has reasons for its food choices. Such communities also have tolerance for others who do not follow their particular regimen.

Many spiritual leaders such as the Buddha, Jesus, and Muhammad were also practical men who realized that the ideal of not killing animals for meat was, for many, difficult to attain. Theravada Buddhist monks usually eat whatever food is offered, even meat. Saint Benedict writes, "Let everyone, except the sick who are very weak, abstain entirely from eating the meat of four-footed animals." In general, the wisdom traditions make allowances for those who have certain health needs.

The example of Jesus, who decided to make all foods "clean," reminds us that the mere fact that someone eats a particular kind of food doesn't define him or her as a good or bad person. The Buddha died at the age of eighty from dysentery caused by a meal of boar's flesh. Hitler was a vegetarian—albeit an unbalanced one, according to *Food and Healing* author Annemarie Colbin.

To look at food the way a monk does, though, means understanding food's ability to nourish the spiritual self and provide deep insight into our actions, feelings, and mind. To accomplish these ends, monks employ one very basic inner meal practice at the spiritual dinner table: mindfulness. This practice is not exclusive of the monastic life. Knowing how to access the power of mindfulness can lead to a life in which every moment becomes sacred and every action is part of our spiritual training ground.

Benefits of the Mindful Meal

If ritual is the appetizer for the spiritual meal, then mindfulness is the main course. Mindfulness often seems elusive and invisible like the air. But it is here, all around us. We only need to summon it by letting go of the mind that looks and examines and analyzes.

To experience mindfulness means surrendering the mind of control, relinquishing the mind of learning, giving up the mind of opinions and desires and expectations. Through this process we find that there is another kind of mind—one steeped in deep observation, receptivity, intent, and action. When mindful eating occurs magic happens, and we cease to dwell on the food itself. What's more, our ego-oriented pattern of eating and desire diminishes.

The mystical *Tao Tê Ching*, from a translation by R.B. Blakney, tells us how to capture the elusive, mindful Way:

> *The student learns by daily increment.*
> *The Way is gained by daily loss,*
> *Loss upon loss until*
> *At last comes rest.*
> *By letting go, it all gets done;*
> *The world is won by those who let it go!*
> *But when you try and try,*
> *The world is then beyond the winning.*

Releasing desires, eliminating habits, and shedding selfishness occur day by day, moment by moment. Eventually, as the mind grows ever more quiet what reveals itself is the inner self and mindfulness of the present moment.

To dwell in the present moment with a sense of serenity and peace— regardless of those inevitable bumps in the road—is one of the advantages of mindfulness. Metaphorically, this is much like the difference between going camping with or without the proper supplies. Without a tent, food, and supplies we may feel unsafe, unprotected, cold, fearful, and hungry. With the right equipment we can enjoy all nature has to offer. Likewise, mindfulness gives us the courage to face each moment at the dinner table with joy, confidence, awareness, caring, understanding, and openness.

Once we manage to peel away the underlying desire for food, what's left is just our body eating and receiving nourishment. And there is just our mind that desires to eat. Through this process we become less and less attached to the foods we eat and the desires they represent. As we develop this kind of clarity, we become better prepared to scan the foods in front of us—whether on a menu or a table—and mindfully choose those that are best.

Mindfulness means tending not only to ourselves, but to others. This is practiced, for example, by offering food and drink to others whenever their plate or glass is empty. Being mindful in these small ways builds our sense of family and community and raises some interesting questions. How often do you acknowledge a waiter or waitress as one who is giving you a blessing? It may be their job, but that doesn't diminish the fact that you are being offered food. By learning to respect this sacred connection, by acting with kindness and gratitude, you can alter any dining experience.

Once we have become mindful, each morsel can be appreciated in completeness, just as Thich Nhat Hanh, in *Our Appointment with Life*, describes for those who drink a cup of tea:

> *When we drink tea in mindfulness, we practice coming back to the present moment to live our life right*

*here. When our mind and our body are fully in the
present moment, then the steaming cup of tea appears
clearly to us. We know it is a wonderful aspect of existence. At that time we are really in contact with the
cup of tea. It is only at times like this that life is really
present.*

Three Steps to Mindfulness

If mindfulness begins with a statement of intention, then it
may be said that preparation and cooking *without* intention lacks
mindfulness. But what really is mindfulness? Is it about being in the
present moment? Is it about doing one thing at a time? Is it about
shifting the focus of our thoughts and attention? Yes, mindfulness is
all these things, but that doesn't really help us *know* it. Mindfulness
is best understood and grasped through its practice, rather than by
a simple definition. Let's start by putting mindfulness into the context of the kitchen. We are going to make a mindful salad.

Suppose you've decided to make a salad. After all, salad is
easy to make, and you've done it many times before—so a mindful
one shouldn't be much of a problem. But on this particular day
there are a thousand other things you'd like to be doing. The sun is
shining and you'd rather be jogging. You are thinking about how
you need to call a business associate. The kids are making a ruckus
in the next room. The phone won't stop ringing. A local news report keeps blaring alarming crime statistics.

As you make your imaginary salad, your mind drifts between
these and other intrusions. That's when the unexpected happens:
things spill, utensils get misplaced, fingers may get cut, and necessary ingredients are missing or improperly measured. Or you slap
the whole thing together as quickly as possible and find you are
totally unaware that you have, in fact, just made a salad.

Step One: Begin with Clear Intention. When problem sce-
narios occur, it may be a sign that your intentions and actions are
not in sync. Or perhaps you never clearly stated your intention in
the first place. Mindfulness begins with intention. Your mindful salad

may begin by stating an intention such as "My intention is to chop lettuce for the salad." This single intention, however, contains many smaller intentions. These could be stated as "I intend to wash the lettuce. I intend to place the lettuce on the cutting board. I intend to lower the knife and cut the lettuce." Each of these intentions precedes an action. If you think that all this slows down the process of chopping lettuce, you're absolutely right! After more practice, though, your intentions will flow, as will the actions that follow them.

Step Two: Follow Through with Action. For mindfulness to work smoothly, intention needs to be followed up by a bodily movement and action. This is really cause and effect: the mind gives the command, and the body follows through with an action. The more deeply intention and action get connected, the closer we are to being in command of the present moment.

Experiencing this kind of mindfulness can be powerful—like seeing a lightning flash and hearing the thunder clap simultaneously. If your mind is typically busy with many thoughts, don't be surprised if you find this new awareness a little unsettling. You are immersed in the moment and you know it. Still, this takes much practice, and there may be times when you forget you even sliced that tomato.

Step Three: Watch and Observe. Mindfulness continues with the step of watching and observing as you follow through with each action—such as actually chopping the lettuce. As you watch and observe, be prepared to shift your attention again and again, all the while observing. This means paying close attention to each part of the entire range of intentions and actions, from beginning to end. When you do this, you place your attention fully on the act of chopping, washing, or cleaning. Observe each movement, allowing yourself to experience it completely. The mindfulness that occurs in this way unfolds through a series of intentions and movements, each occurring in successive moments that only feel and seem continuous.

Pausing before changing intentions and actions is important in mindfulness, because it helps us focus on the one thing we are doing at that moment. In *Wisdom Distilled From The Daily*, Joan Chittister writes: "In addition to silence, community customs, and the common table, the monastic practices of *statio* and *lectio* are also tools of the spiritual craft. *Statio* is a monastic custom that was born centuries ago but clearly belongs in this one. *Statio* is the practice of stopping one thing before we begin another. It is the time between times." As such, *statio* is useful practice at the dinner table, or to center oneself before any activity.

As you watch and observe, have compassion for yourself. If you happen to drop something, move too quickly, become distracted, or even find yourself feeling frustrated by the slow pace, that's okay. Just gently return to your mindful moment. With practice and patience, you cannot help but succeed.

Mindful Preparation

There is a story about an elderly Zen Buddhist *tenzo*, or cook, who was drying mushrooms in the scorching sun. When the cook was asked why he didn't have an assistant, he replied, "No one else is me." This story illustrates how kitchen work is more than a responsibility in helping to prepare a meal for others. It is a personal practice that helps us stay on the inner meal path. By mindfully preparing and cooking a meal, we also cook our inner selves.

This mindful approach to preparation is not exclusive to Zen and Buddhism. There comes to mind Saint Ignatius, founder of the Jesuit order in the sixteenth century, who exalted the concept of finding God through life's daily experiences. Part of his prescribed spiritual practice includes an "Examen of Conscience," or a daily self-examination of one's relationship with God and others.

As Jesuit Brother Rick Curry illustrates in *The Secrets of Jesuit Breadmaking*, the secret of breadmaking—or any kitchen work—begins by adding a spiritual ingredient:

> *When I make bread, I make an Examen of Conscience. After reading the recipe, I take a deep breath, relax, and recall that I am in God's presence. I recall the last twenty-four hours and name the good things that have come into my life, and I thank God for them. After the*

*dough has been mixed and begins to rise, I reflect on
how I have participated in this new life, and I beg God
to show me how I am growing more alive in my spiritual life. I examine what my recent actions, omissions,
thoughts, and desires tell me about my relationship to
God and myself and others in God. I examine how I
have dealt with my family and coworkers. Have I spent
any time in the last twenty-four hours doing something
generous for another? Do I harbor resentment? Have I
held my tongue? Have I prayed for another's needs? Has
my conversation been hurtful? Am I part of the problem
or part of the solution? Have I been kind? Have I remembered that God is lovingly watching over me?"*

Where does mindfulness in preparation begin? Where does it
end? Ancient texts like *The Rule of Saint Benedict* and *Instructions
for the Zen Cook* by Zen Master Dogen—written in the sixth and
thirteenth centuries, respectively—still guide many monasteries in
details of how to care for and clean utensils, as well as how to
manage the kitchen. These texts have endured because what they say
works, especially within the context of the family and community.

For example, Saint Benedict describes the duties of monks,
from the monastery cellarer, who "will regard all utensils and goods
of the monastery as sacred vessels of the altar," to the brothers who
"should serve one another. Consequently, no one will be excused
from kitchen service unless he is sick or engaged in some important
business for the monastery, for such service increases reward and
fosters love."

What Saint Benedict means is that by taking part in meal
preparation and by serving each other, we elevate the entire work-
ings of the kitchen into the spiritual realm. At the same time, we
make a declaration of love and caring for ourselves and others.

There are many ways to manifest Saint Benedict's sentiments.
For example, do you offer to lend a hand when you're invited to
someone's house for dinner? Do you help clean up after a party?

Does each member of your family have a responsibility at mealtime? By not taking part in kitchen activities, we may be depriving ourselves of an opportunity to advance on our journey along inner our meal path.

Each action—cleaning utensils, choosing ingredients, handling food, and cooking—can be done with full attention and awareness. To accomplish this requires letting go of the rational mind and allowing the power of the moment to fill us up. Whenever this happens we feel our aliveness, with all our senses able to operate freely and clearly. Simply by stating our intention to bring attention and focus to a meal, we are like the Zen cook who, according to Zen Master Dogen, "tries to build great temples from ordinary greens." Food—because of its life-sustaining nature—is a natural doorway into the state of mindfulness. To enter, we need only to awaken to the moment.

Mindfulness Practice

Practicing mindfulness can at first seem a bit daunting. I am reminded, in particular, of a meal that took place during the retreat at which I was first initiated. As I enter the dining room at 11 A.M., a monk motions for me to sit directly opposite from the Sayadaw, or abbot. I straighten my robes and take a seat on an old wooden, straight-backed chair and try to squeeze my long legs under the low table. Glancing across the table at the Venerable U Silananda—a well-known teacher and author of *The Four Foundations of Mindfulness*—I momentarily worry about not being mindful enough. But soon I forget all about that and, while eating in silence, simply practice intention, movement, and observation. The silence helps me filter out distractions and allows for greater concentration and mindfulness.

I notice the Sayadaw eats moderately. I slow down my eating, consciously raising the food to my mouth, feeling gratitude for each bite. I try to pause before each movement, first stating whatever my intention is. There are many: to choose the food I want, to reach for the food with the fork, to raise it up to my mouth, to chew, to taste, to swallow, and to hand orange slices to another monk, and so on.

At the same time, I observe all the thoughts that pass through my mind. These include my enjoying the taste, my desiring more food, my craving for another kind of food, and my being distracted and looking around the table. I try not to dwell on the food, but rather to place my attention on the intent, the action, and the observation of the action and thoughts that arise. As often as my mind wanders, I gently bring it back to mindfulness.

At one point during the lunch, a young girl, the daughter of the family that offered our meal, holds out a small cake. She smiles shyly as the Sayadaw receives it from her and places it on the table. I am astonished that I have no taste for anything sweet and moist like this cake. The mealtime's mindfulness has let me deeply observe my food desires and habits—much like opening up a wristwatch to see what makes it tick. Mindfulness splinters my usual habits and patterns, allowing me to select a more balanced choice of foods.

Later that night, not only am I not hungry, but that notorious Cadbury's milk chocolate bar becomes less and less of a temptation. I know, of course, that my sense desires aren't just going to disappear. But I feel a certain comfort in knowing that my desires are balanced by my mindfulness and awareness.

Mindfulness is available to us all, right here, right now. It is one of life's most important seasonings. After all, mindfulness cultivates freedom of choice that both nourishes and satisfies the soul. For as the Venerable U Silananda once told me, "Mindfulness is free. We are born with it."

PRACTICE: FINDING YOUR HUNGRY GHOST

Are you a hungry ghost? The Tibetan Book of the Dead —written in the fourteenth century—discloses the various realms said to exist after death. The soul must confront these realms in order to reach nirvana, or bliss. Yet in another sense, these realms can be thought of as existing on the earthly plane as well. The realm of the hungry ghost, for instance, is one of desire, possession, and hunger. In life, this may manifest as a state of mind and an approach to living.

The image of the hungry ghost is that of someone with an enormous stomach, a very slender neck, and a tiny mouth. The problem with hungry ghosts is this: they never get enough of what they desire. They can never fill the hunger in their giant belly. In fact, having more only creates an even greater desire. Imagine for a minute an insatiable desire for food so great that you continue to crave it even after you have gorged so much that you can't eat another bite. But there's no more joy, only pain in trying to possess more and more of that which you can never get enough of.

To some degree, we all experience the deprivation of hungry ghosts when our needs aren't met. Mindfulness is one tool for helping ease the pain of food's hungry ghosts. Use this exercise whenever you feel you need to practice self-observation or prepare yourself for mindfulness.

Do this reflection immediately before going to eat. Spend a few minutes visiting a local fast-food restaurant or an all-you-can-eat buffet. Even if you normally never eat at that particular establishment, go inside and just observe nonjudgmentally. Try to imagine that this is the first time you have ever been to a restaurant. In fact, try to imagine that you don't even know what purpose food serves. Do you notice any hungry ghosts or find much mindfulness among the patrons?

It is possible that, from your new vantage point of mindfulness and awareness of spiritual eating, you may perceive food and eating as never before. The point of this exercise isn't to feel superior to those who eat poorly or who live as hungry ghosts led about by their hunger for food. Rather, it is to let you feel a sense of compassion, understanding, and loving-kindness for those with a particular way of eating.

Slowly, allow yourself to become aware of your own hungry ghost. Listen to its hunger and cries for more attention. Don't repress or ignore what you hear, but instead feed your hungry ghost with love and mindfulness. After you have finished observing, sit down for your own meal—at a restaurant where you can be nourished with healthy food. Now, with compassion for yourself and others, practice mindfulness during your meal. Try to remember that the desires, cravings, feelings of guilt, and other thoughts you may experience do not define you. Simply acknowledge your thoughts and return to your mindfulness.

Finding our hungry ghost offers many benefits. It exposes the kind of hunger that fast-food restaurants cater to. It helps us uncover our hidden desires. It lets us experience what it is like to eat in a mindful and aware manner.

PRACTICE: MINDFUL BREATHING

Mindful breathing is a good way to anchor the practice of mindfulness. In addition, breathing is a natural antidote to anxiety and stress. In the 1970s, cardiologist and researcher Herbert Benson found that meditation and other breathing techniques created what he called "the relaxation response." The relaxation response has been well documented. Because this response cools down and calms the body—by lowering metabolism, heart rate, and blood pressure—it is often useful for pain management, relief from depression, and anxiety.

The exercise that follows will not only establish a good foundation for mindfulness, it will help relax you as well!

When you take a breath, do you breathe into your chest or into your diaphragm? Mindful diaphragmatic breathing is the best way to experience the benefits of relaxation. That's why you first need to differentiate between chest breathing and diaphragmatic breathing, or belly breathing. While seated, place one hand on your chest and the other hand on your belly—just below the rib cage. Now breath normally. Be aware of what rises and falls: the belly or the chest? Or both?

If only your chest rises, then you are breathing shallowly. Chest breathing activates the body's alert system. For example, if you were under stress or a state of alarm, this would be a normal place to breath. However, many people breath here when it's not necessary.

If your abdomen rises and falls while breathing, then you are breathing more deeply into your lungs. This automatically activates your body's relaxation system. If you find it difficult to breath into your belly, try cupping your hands behind your head. This will open the rib cage and make belly breathing easier. Once you know what this feels like, you can lower your arms to your side or place them in your lap while practicing.

After a moment of centering, mentally state your intention to create an in-breath. Follow up your intention by breathing into your diaphragm. Take a normal in-breath, and as you do, observe the rise of your abdomen. Take a brief pause, and mentally state your intention to end a breath. Follow up on this intention by breathing out slowly and observing how your abdomen falls. Repeat your in-breath and out-breath with intention, action, and observation. If thoughts intrude, just return to your mindful breathing. After this comes more naturally, you may want to drop the mental intention and just breath—still being mindful of your readiness to create a breath and to end a breath.

One variation is to take deeper breaths. To do this, set the intention to create a long in-breath and to end a long breath. This will increase your mindful concentration and focus. As you do this, just breath a little deeper and longer. Let mindful breathing work for you. Use it often, while standing in line or whenever you need a mindful moment.

12 – Empty Stomach, Full Spirit

You have reproved me for eating
very little,
but I only eat to live,
whereas you live to eat.

— Socrates

On a recent predawn morning at the cottage I step outside. I am greeted only by a lone star twinkling brightly in the eastern sky— could it be Venus? At this early hour, the depth of silence from the surrounding neighborhood gives space to other sounds. Birds— hundreds of them, I imagine—chirp, tweet, warble, caw, and twit- ter in ways I've never heard, creating a remarkable orchestral score.

The dim, throaty roar of a freight train echoes in the far-off darkness. The silhouette of palm trees rises against dawn's blank canvas. And I walk. One step, foot rising, moving forward, touching ground. Shoe tops soaked from the dew. In the darkness, there is only one lone star above. Only one lone person walking below. One step. One step. One step at a time.

It strikes me that fasting is like a solitary walk under the stars. We alone must take that first step. Here, we step onto a path of self-discovery. Here, we aspire to reach for and experience something beyond the ordinary. Here, through diligence and effort we hope to glimpse our true self. It is comforting to know that while a fast is ours alone, this path has been trodden by many others before us.

The word *fasting* conjures up many associations—positive and negative—that tell us a lot about how we feel toward renunciation, discipline, desire, craving, control, and other aspects of our lives. The unusual and often amazing tales that populate this subject include those of the Hindu practice of *prayopavesha*, or self-willed death by fasting; the Korean Buddhist monk who has not eaten in three years, taking nourishment only from natural spring water and by raising his palms upward to receive energy from the sun at noontime; the Eskimo women who undertake petitionary fasts when their mates go hunting for food; the medieval women, obsessed with fasting, whose bodies were believed to nevertheless secrete oils, milks, and other life-sustaining liquids; and the dramatic political fasts of Gandhi, who learned fasting from his mother.

Fasts have been practiced for thousands of years. The historian Philo described one sect of Jewish ascetics—influenced by Greek philosophy and known as the Therapeutae—that lived over two thousand years ago and embraced prolonged fasting. Karl Suso Frank, in *With Greater Liberty*, writes: "In the hellenistic world, it was, above all, philosophical schools that taught emphatically ascetical regimens. They took the concept 'asceticism' out of its original context—the artisan's skill and the athlete's training—and transferred it to the context of human spiritual perfection."

Over time, pagan rituals of purification and renunciation became accepted within the broader cultural and religious context. This was especially true of early Christians, who adapted Jewish fasts for their own use. Jesus had previously set many examples of renunciation for Christians to follow. With the stage thus set, Christianity adopted the ascetic life as one of its tenets—and in doing so gained what was considered to be an important philosophical approach to life.

In Medieval times, fasting gained greater significance. Lenten and weekly fasts became a yardstick of piety. Yet fasting may have signified more than just devotion. At a time when famine threatened and gluttony was considered as lust, renouncing food may have been a means to attain even a small measure of control over one's life.

How important was food during the Middle Ages? According to Caroline Walker Bynum, the author of *Holy Feast and Holy Fast*, food served as the ultimate status symbol. The mark of aristocratic privilege was "gorging and vomiting, [and] luxuriating in food." In fact, to voluntarily give up food or feed others was a major sacrifice, if not a saintly and courageous deed. This was especially true for women, who possessed little power or control over their lives. If certain practices gave them back control over their bodies, as well as spiritual nourishment, then the incentive to use food as a means of personal power became that much greater.

As history shows, the desire for food and the need to exercise control over its intake have always been at odds. Even today, we feel this pressure in many subtle and not so subtle ways. Sometimes it's helpful to recognize and give a face to these pressures by asking a few questions. What are the first foods that greet me when I enter the supermarket? Is it true that diet books are located near the checkout counter? How many food-related commercials and advertisements did I see today? How many advertisements for health, fitness, and dieting? How often during the day do thoughts about food enter my mind? As your capacity for spiritual eating grows, you may be surprised at the answers to these questions.

Since food serves as the basis for our survival, it comes as no surprise that it is often on our minds. But when does simply thinking about it or planning our next meal turn into an obsession?

Awareness is one of the keys to spiritual eating and freedom from craving, obsession, and addiction. When we are unaware of our thoughts and our desires, we can be stretched like a rubber band between food control on one side and food lust on the other.

I remember noticing, on a recent visit to a bookstore, that the diet books and cookbooks were positioned directly opposite each other in the same aisle. It actually makes a lot of sense. If we're obsessed with food at all, we will always be faced with an ongoing struggle and the question, Which way to turn?

Benefits of Fasting

What does all this have to do with fasting? Fasting, when used properly, can help bring into balance the two opposing food pressures. What follows are the benefits and advantages of what I like to call a compassionate and moderate fast. Such a fast can build up the awareness, strength, and self-discipline with which we approach food. It gives our stomachs a rest from time to time and helps cleanse our bodies. It helps us realize how dependent we are on food and the Earth that provides us with sustenance. It humbles us with the realization of what hunger feels like. It lets us appreciate the wondrous gift of life and consciousness. It lets us know what it means to sacrifice something of value. It improves our mental concentration and focus. It reminds us not to be selfish. It makes us more aware of our own "hungry ghosts" of greed and envy. It teaches us the value of charity. It alters our consciousness by letting us practice patience and nonattachment. It empowers us to break long-lived habits. It binds us to our commitments. It improves our ability to discriminate between those foods that are best for us and those that are not. It lets us surrender our passions. It encourages compassion for our needs and the needs of other human beings. It allows us to experience the sense of peace that comes from being free from desire. Not least of all, it helps us transcend our physical being and puts us in touch with our spiritual self.

For many of us, fasting is experienced on a special occasion—usually as an anchor of spiritual preparation before a festival. The fasting found in wisdom traditions tends toward moderation. Most Biblical fasts occur only on special occasions and last no more than a day. Even Islam's lengthy, twenty-nine-day Ramadan fast allows food between the times of sunset and sunrise. In contrast, the famous fasts of those like Moses, Jesus, Elijah, Buddha, and Gandhi are truly extraordinary. Still, this powerful mindful practice, when approached with compassion and moderation, offers something for everyone.

The traditional reasons for fasting are many—spiritual, petitionary, self-denial, therapeutic, political, penitential, mourning, and religious. Used in these ways, fasting becomes a tool for inner growth.

Native American tribes, for example, commonly use fasting during the sacred sweat ceremony, or sweat lodge. Stones are first heated in a fire pit until red-hot, then placed in the center of a closed hut or dome. This rite of cleansing and purification—usually accompanied with prayer and song—prepares the participant for a marriage, a vision quest, or another sacred ceremony. In *Native American Mythology*, Page Bryant writes: "The Sweat is not an endurance test. It is the womb of *Mother Earth*, the place where Native people go to cleanse and renew themselves and to be reborn."

In the Jewish tradition, fasting and prayer combine during the High Holy Day of Yom Kippur, or the Day of Atonement. During this twenty-four-hour period, Jews admit their sins and sit in judgment of their past year's actions. Just as giving up food purifies the physical being, admitting and atoning for sins purifies the spiritual.

In addition to occasional fasts, many wisdom traditions also use periodic fasts to accomplish less specific goals, but goals that are nevertheless just as important. For Hindus, fasting is an ethical practice. As Swami Prabhavananda writes in *The Spiritual Heritage of India*, "The ultimate moral ideal of the Upanisads is complete self-abnegation, the utter renunciation of all selfish and personal desires." Members of Paramahansa Yogananda's Hindu-oriented Self-Realization Fellowship, for example, fast once a week to allow the body to rest. Shutting down the metabolism frees up energy for meditation that is normally used for digestion.

The Hindu mystic Shankara tells us that by transcending the physical we can gain self-liberation and knowledge of our inner self:

Who is bound?
He who is attached to worldliness.

How is heaven attained?
The attainment of heaven is freedom from cravings.

What destroys craving?
Realization of one's true self.

Who are our enemies?
Our sense-organs, when they are uncontrolled.

Who are our friends?
Our sense-organs, when they are controlled.

Who has overcome the world?
He who has conquered his own mind.

—Shankara, from *Crest - Jewel of Discrimination*,
translated by Swami Prabhavananda and Christopher
Isherwood

For Buddhists of the Theravadan tradition, periodic fasting is
part of the larger practice of self-discipline. With fasting comes the
observance of nine precepts for proper conduct, as well as meditation. Periodic fast days also connect followers to the rhythms of
nature and the moon, which means a fast approximately once every
eight days.

The precepts are repeated on the morning of the fast day.
The participant vows to act in accordance with the following activities: to refrain from killing any living being, to refrain from taking
what is not given, to refrain from incelibacy, to refrain from false
speech, to refrain from any drinks and drugs that reduce mindfulness, to refrain from taking food after noon, to refrain from partaking in luxury, to refrain from any form of entertainment, and, finally,

to transmit infinite amounts of loving-kindness to all beings regardless of religion or race.

A Compassionate and Moderate Fast

Fasting is not a panacea that magically removes toxins from our body or eliminates our food and diet problems. It is, however, a powerful tool for advancing us along the road to self-discovery, conscious awareness, and spiritual transcendence. Bearing in mind that we are not machines, we can't simply undergo a fast—which causes a drastic change in our diet—in the same casual way that we send our car in for a tune-up or an oil change.

According to my dictionary, the word *fast* is defined as "to abstain from eating all or certain foods." Because fasting is not by definition a normally moderate action, we need to introduce compassion. We can begin to show compassion for ourselves by listening—to our bodies and to others—for feedback on our fasting methods. Above all, do not take this practice lightly. Always seek medical advice from a doctor and nutritionist.

Personally, I had never really fasted in any meaningful way—except for the once-yearly Yom Kippur fast while growing up—until I began my practice of regular daily fasting as a monk. Though I still practice my "monk's fast" one day a week, I try not to be rigid with it. If I feel tired or weak, I let my intuition guide me whether or not to break the fast. This is, after all, a way of showing compassion toward myself.

The purpose of fasting is not to set any endurance records. By introducing moderation into a fast, you show concern and caring for your body, mind, and spirit. Moderation also shows good judgment and an appreciation for the feelings of those closest to you. Since fasting restricts food intake, you can enhance the success of a fast by eating a balanced meal beforehand. It may also be useful to practice some form of centering prayer or reflection with your fast. As Jesus and others have shown, fasts are easier to maintain when combined with prayer.

The guidelines for your compassionate and moderate fast can be determined by asking questions, such as: What kind of a fast is best for me? What are my reasons for fasting? What do I hope to accomplish by fasting?

Deciding to go without food is to make a commitment to personal liberation—from the demands of desire, craving, and attachment. Yet because fasting is personal, the length of a fast, what foods to restrict, and how to endow it with meaning are entirely your choice. Some people fast exclusively for health reasons, others for spiritual practice.

Use the inner meal exercise at the end of this chapter to lead you more securely onto this useful, though sometimes misunderstood, road. Remember, though, that even Buddha—as translated in the *Dhammapada* by Byrom—cautions those who fast without understanding the bigger picture:

> *For months the fool may fast,*
> *Eating from the tip of a grass blade.*
> *Still he is not worth a penny*
> *Beside the master whose food*
> *is the way.*

After the Fast

I can still remember one of my first "break-fast" meals at the monastery. On this particular day, I awaken at 3:45 A.M. to the sound of distant thunder. Quietly, I make my bed and walk to the meditation room—guided only by a low-wattage night light. I practice walking meditation until 5 A.M., when I join seven monks for an hour and a half of sitting meditation.

We sit, cloaked in the dark and stillness, when, without warning, it begins to pour. Sheets of rain pound at the roof, and before long, water gushes from the gutters onto the ground in the courtyard. Finally, the rain abates, and the storm soon diminishes into a shower, then into a trickle. The appetite, I think to myself, can sometimes act upon us with as much force and suddenness as a cloudburst. Fasting, strangely enough, can reduce even a thunderous appetite to a drizzle.

At 6:30 A.M. I sit down for breakfast. It dawns on me that although I've been up since early that morning, I am still not hungry. Even while fasting the entire day and night before I suffered no pangs of hunger.

But now, I am face to face with steaming bowls of a Burmese soup consisting of noodles, fish, lemon grass, ginger, garlic, crunchy chick peas, red chile peppers, and a dash of fresh-squeezed lemon. Also offered are oatmeal and raisins, hot croissants, yogurt, grapefruit, bananas, almonds, and some pound cake.

Having gone without food for some time, I wonder whether I can eat moderately, or if my food-deprived appetite will respond to the breakfast feast with a thunderous, cloudburst-like rumble. I decide to try a technique one of the monks has told me about—that of scanning the table to intuitively sense which foods my body needs.

I also decide to follow the lead of some of the monks and wait for all the food to be placed on the table before eating. As it turns out, the act of pausing mindfully lets me sense and feel my hunger. It allows me to recognize the strength of my desire without immediately giving in to it. This, in turn, helps me build resistance and keeps me from eating what my body doesn't really need. To my surprise, these simple methods of scanning and waiting work, allowing me to eat slowly, moderately, and mindfully.

Personally, I like to use these methods when baskets of chips or other snacks are placed on the table prior to a meal. By waiting, I'm not denying or controlling my desire for a particular food. In fact, I'm doing just the opposite—I'm giving myself total freedom and permission to eat that snack, but only *after* all the food arrives. When snacks are the only food on the table, my mind's desire to eat attaches completely to that one food source. But when desire for food is spread equally among a wide variety of foods, snacks are rarely all that tempting. In reality, I'm just giving myself the opportunity to make a more informed decision—one that benefits my body and spirit.

These simple methods are available to us all—whether or not we are ending a fast. Try them, and you may find that moderation and healthy eating become a regular part of your spiritual diet.

Feasting—A Communal Path

No exploration of fasting would be complete without looking at the origins of the feast. Feasts and festivals serve as bookends to the fast, giving us an important container for our communal celebrations and emotions. Festivals let us honor major life passages—births, weddings, initiations, and deaths—and can be celebrated in the home, in a place of worship, or with the community. In many cultures and traditions, festivals also bring meaning to the rhythms of nature, the death and birth of the seasons, eclipses, and other movements of the moon and sun. Most importantly, festivals let us give and receive food as an expression of our joy, caring, and the fact that we exist in an interconnected web of life.

While some festivals, like Judaism's *Rosh Hashanah*, or New Year, precede a fast, most follow one. It's the anticipation created during fasting that makes any feast that much more special. Both Lent and Ramadan are powerful examples of how fasting and feasting are joined, each enabling the other to exist to its fullest potential.

Christianity's observance of Lent—which dates back to the fourth century—recalls the temptation Jesus faced during his forty days in the wilderness. It requires followers to fast or renounce a luxury for an equal number of days. This is done as spiritual preparation for the Easter Sunday feast and the celebration of Jesus' resurrection.

Islam's month long Ramadan fast culminates with the *Eid-ul Fitr*, or fast-breaking feast. On this day fasting is strictly forbidden, as *Eid-ul Fitr* commemorates the hardship and sacrifice of the prior fast as well as gratefulness to God.

Ritual feasts gain much of their meaning from the particular season or crop with which they are associated. Even today, for example, it is easy to forget how much of the world still depends on monsoon rains for crop production. Ritual feasts permit us—whether we are part of a tribe or a community—to encounter those powers or deities that bridge the vagaries and uncertainties of nature and survival.

The green corn dance of Native Americans, for example, traditionally celebrates the first crop of the new season. India's festivals for wheat and rice, as described by Gene Spiller and Rowena

Hubbard in *Nutrition Secrets of the Ancients*, arrive like clockwork with the harvest:

> *In the northern Punjab, the traditional festival of Baisakhi celebrates the wheat harvest with music, dancing, and abundant food. In the southern states, Pongal, the three-day rice festival, was celebrated with ox-cart races and foods made from the newly harvested rice.*

Other harvest festivals of thanksgiving, such as the Jewish Sukkot, or Feast of Booths, find their basis in scripture. "You shall keep the feast of booths seven days...[and] you shall rejoice in your feast," states the Bible in Deuteronomy. Throughout this festive, seven-day period, rectangular booths—each known as a *sukkah*—are made and decorated with palms, fruit, vegetables, and other greenery and foodstuffs. Families invite their friends to join them under the sukkah to eat meals and sleep under the stars. Festivals such as this bring its followers another step closer to nature's sustaining touch. When used in this way, festivals can help us shift out of the world of worry and material needs and into nature's timeless spectacle.

Ritual feasts also make sense out of the loss of life, fertility, and even food production caused by Earth's seasonal shifts. The ancient Egyptian autumn festival, which marked Osiris' death, coincided with the beginning of winter and the changing level of the River Nile. Celtic pagan feasts like All Saints and All Souls Day—later adopted by Christianity—originally commemorated the passing of summer and the dawning of winter. Even today, the centuries-old Japanese Obon festival continues to pay homage to ancestral spirits through dance, prayer, and lanterns floated on water to light the way for the soul to follow on its visit home for a waiting meal. For many traditions, midnight ceremonial fires and special food prepared for the arriving spirits are common ingredients.

Festivals make up our common heritage. And, as evident in an ancient song found in J. C. Cooper's *The Dictionary of Festivals*—festivals let us revel in the joy and music of life:

Soul, soul, for a soul cake.
I pray, good mistress, a soul cake,
An apple, or pear, a plum, or a cherry,
Any good thing to make us merry.
One for Peter, two for Paul,
Three for Him who made us all.
Up with the kettle, down with the pan,
Give us good cheer and we'll be gone.

PRACTICE: FASTING

All of us have previous experience with fasting. Even without trying, we practice it each night from the time we fall asleep until the time that we break-fast in the morning. Isn't it ironic that a word we take for granted as representing our morning meal really means to "break the fast"? Still, a daytime fast represents a major departure from our normal eating patterns.

There are no right or wrong answers to the question of why people fast. Fasting is a process of self-discovery. It may even break down old eating habits and free up your approach to food. You may find, for example, that fasting—even on a limited basis—will lead you toward a healthier and more balanced diet. Once shifting into this new mode of spiritual eating, there may no longer be a need for enforcing "food control" in your life.

Fasting, to be deeply and spiritually nourishing, requires a purpose and a strong commitment. Try to reflect on the questions that follow. They may help you develop a better understanding of what benefits a fast can have for you.

What do I want to accomplish with my fast? What is motivating me? Is there a religious fast that I can take part in to help ground me in my commitment? What do I hope to learn through the experience? Do I expect that a fast will be difficult? What will I do if I cannot maintain my fast? How can I fast with compassion and moderation? What form of prayer, reflection, or sacred reading can I use to accompany my fast?

Write down all your answers. Not only will you begin to develop a fast that is right for you, but you may discover the root cause behind your desire to fast. For some, this might be the hidden need to gain control over food. There are short-term and long-term reasons for fasting. What are yours?

When you reflect upon what fast best accommodates you, bear in mind the words *moderate* and *compassionate*. For some, fasting means restricting only certain foods while eating others. Some eat only raw fruits and vegetables during their fasting period. Others may only drink juice and water. Fasts can last for hours, for a day, or even longer. Always make allowances for physical activity, which increases the need for food. Above all, remember that fasting is not an endurance contest.

A compassionate and moderate fast provides many personal benefits. It makes us aware of possibilities for fasting that are unique and suited only to us. It puts us in touch with our personal, internal rhythms. It contributes to our process of self-discovery. It helps us break rigid habits and lets us treat ourselves with compassion. It builds up our resistance to harmful foods. As we establish a new relationship to food, we better appreciate its value and begin to eat a better diet. It generates spiritual energy, effort, and concentration.

KEEP A FASTING DIARY

Maintain a record of the details of your fast. This is an opportunity to write down the insights that you will gain as you go about your daily life without food as a constant distraction. The purpose of fasting is not to be extreme. There's no good done by replacing out-of-control eating with out-of-control fasting. Rather, the purpose is to learn balance and bring perspective to what may be out of balance.

Part Three

RETURN TO SOURCE

13 – The Good, the Bad, the Forbidden

Do you know that trees talk?
Well, they do.
They talk to each other,
and they'll talk to you if you listen....
I have learned a lot from trees:
sometimes about the weather,
sometimes about animals,
sometimes about the Great Spirit.

—Walking Buffalo (Canadian Stoney Indian),
Catch the Whisper of the Wind

Just as the living Earth speaks to the primal traditions, foods talk directly to us—of health, healing, nutrition, and spirit. The wisdom traditions provide us timeless guidelines with a holistic approach to food and the mindful diet. They tell us of common sense do's and don'ts that build upon the experience of countless peoples, cultures, and traditions. While the reasoning behind food choices may differ, the choices themselves often fit into astoundingly similar patterns.

This chapter gives us an opportunity to reflect upon our own food preferences while being tolerant and nonjudgmental toward the choices of others. It is easy to defend our own particular habits as if they were a part of us. Yet by being open to others, we can more fully embrace our own struggles—such as whether or not to eat certain foods—with a greater measure of compassion and understanding.

Over the years, we have become more enlightened as to the effects of air pollution on the environment and our health. Food, like the air, sustains us. In many cultures it serves not only as nourishment, but as medicine that engenders good health, healing, and longevity. There is growing evidence, for example, that beta carotene—an antioxidant found in fruits and vegetables—may prevent cancer. The ancient Chinese belief that tea—especially green tea—possesses healing properties that lower high blood pressure, help prevent cancer, and fight disease is being confirmed in various studies. Even the Food and Drug Administration allows health claims to be made that whole oat bran's soluble fiber "may reduce the risk of heart disease."

In *Spontaneous Healing*, Dr. Andrew Weil devotes a full chapter to what he calls "A Healing Diet." He writes: "Of all the choices we make, those concerning food are particularly important, because we have great potential control over them." His "Healing Diet" uses some commonsense concepts that make food part of one's overall health program. In general, these include such things as reducing overall caloric content, limited or periodic fasting, and ingestion of unprocessed "vegetable oils that are predominantly mono-unsaturated—olive, canola, peanut, avocado"—while reducing intake of saturated animal fats, whole milk products, and "unnatural sources of saturated fat: Margarine, solid vegetable shortening, and all processed foods made with partially hydrogenated oils." He also suggests eating more fruits, vegetables, whole grains, and fish high in omega-3 fatty acids.

If there are questions about this commonsense approach, we need only glimpse back in history. The longevity of ancient Greeks

like Pythagoras, Plato, and others who primarily ate uncooked vegetarian meals with fruits, vegetables, whole grains, and olive oil
makes us wonder—Does the proper diet provide a natural immu-
nity from disease and aging?

Andrew Weil is not alone in making food choices part of an
overall holistic strategy of increasing our awareness of the innate
healing capabilities of our body and spirit. In *Food and Healing*,
Annemarie Colbin writes: "A holistic view of the human body recognizes that its function is affected by a variety of factors, both
internal and external, such as food, drink, exercise, emotions, stress,
and so on. It recognizes that disease symptoms express a total condition of the organism." In other words, we are greater than the sum
of our individual parts. In light of this, how can any nutritional, diet,
or medical system that reduces us into a number of mechanical
parts, either physically or emotionally, truly heal or create balance
within our whole being? Mindful eating, as recommended by the
wisdom traditions, acknowledges this wholeness.

Hinduism—Food for Healing

Though approaching food from distinct cultural and global
perspectives, the wisdom traditions offer us an impressive accumu-
lation of human knowledge about food, spirituality, and health. Hindus believe that all food possesses different properties—*sattva, rajas*, and *tamas*—that affect our body, awareness, and spirit. In this
context, a mindful diet is critical—because to consume a food is to
consume its energy characteristic. In other words, the vibrational
and chemical makeups of our bodies are altered by the foods we
ingest.

Vegetarian eating, for example, is preferred over meat—because of the negative karmic energy that arises from the act of killing. For example, tamasic-based foods such as the meat and by-
products of cows and pigs, as well as fermented foods, alcohol, and
other mind altering substances, harm the body and contain static
properties that cause inertia, laziness, weakness, and hinder a desire for spiritual growth. Rajasic-based foods such as caffeine, choco-

late, tea, curry, and other hot spices—as well as less damaging animal foods like fowl, fish, lamb, and eggs—contain stimulating properties that cause excess emotion, action, agitation, and ambition. Sattvic-based foods such as fresh fruits, beans, sprouted seeds, whole grains, mainly raw vegetables, pure juices, milk and dairy products, honey, and certain spices and herbs contain enlightening properties that cause sentience, balance, and clarity.

A sophisticated system of traditional Indian medicine called *Ayurveda*, which in Sanskrit means "the science of life," is practiced in India and steeped in Hindu concepts and methods. In the most general terms, this holistic form of medicine uses diet, nontoxic herbs and oils, meditation, yoga, exercise, and other therapies to bring the body's three humors, or bio-energies, into balance. Because these humors correspond to bodily functions and organs, healthy life becomes a matter of maintaining the balance of our energy.

The concept of "food combining"—popular in many diets—has long been a part of Ayurvedic practice. When it comes to food choices, our life-sustaining energy achieves balance through a complex system of food combinations, the season, the time of day, whether a food is cooked or raw, and even our emotional state. All food impacts on the energies that coexist within us. Wholesome food—such as rice, carrots, peas, and grapes—digests easily, keeps the body's humors in balance, provides energy for both body and mind, and opens up the body's energy pathways. Unwholesome food, however, is not always necessarily bad. While some foods may block the body's energy or be hard to digest, they can still be included in the diet if eaten in combination with other foods, especially the proper herbs and spices.

Since the right food combination makes all the difference to health, it's just as important to avoid antagonistic combinations. Foods that are antagonistic—either to one another or the time of year—may act as a toxin and should never be eaten. In *Ayurveda for Life*, Dr. Vinod Verma gives examples of antagonistic foods, such as: "Milk with sour things...Honey with wine...Not eating according to seasons, such as eating nuts in summer, cold drinks in winter, etc....[and]...Not eating according to the geographic location."

According to the Ayurvedic system, each of us is unique, and everything we do—how we breathe, the foods we eat, where we live, and what we think—exerts a profound influence on our whole being. Here we find two common themes that appear across the wisdom traditions: a tolerance for personal differences and the acknowledgment that whole, local, and seasonal foods contain special value. In essence, foods that elevate and enhance the spirit also promote good health and longevity, while those which harm the spirit reduce health and injure the body. This is all the more reason to find a mindful and spiritual diet that soothes not just one part of us, but the whole soul.

Buddhism and Taoism—Food for Long Life

As with Hinduism's ancient Ayurvedic nutrition, Buddhism and Taoism impact our modern eating habits through a variety of holistic approaches. One cornerstone of Buddhism's mindful diet comes from the Buddha's advice against killing any sentient being for a meal, taking food unjustly, or taking food by force. Many Buddhists bring themselves into balance and harmony with life and nature through what is traditionally a vegetarian diet. In general, whole, seasonal foods are preferred to those that are refined, processed, canned, and preserved.

Zen Buddhism uses a philosophy of cooking that speeds spiritual development and total health. This style of vegetable cooking—known as *shojin ryori*—originated in China and was transplanted to Japan by monks. In *The Elements of Zen*, authors David Scott and Tony Doubleday state that "the underlying principle of shojin ryori is the very simple one of love and gratitude for the food received. Preparing and partaking of food becomes part of the religious practice and takes its place alongside other contributions to the happiness and welfare of society and ourselves."

Mindful diet was almost an obsession for ancient Taoist longevity and vitality cults. They accumulated knowledge of nutrition, herbs, breathing, acupuncture, and the polarities of yin/yang—all toward the purpose of attaining and augmenting *ch'i*, life's vital energy that is stored in our bodies. Today, traditional Chinese medicine uses many of these ideas, especially the belief that balanced energy flow through the body's meridian channels makes for good health.

A mindful diet contains energy that helps build up *ch'i*. This bolsters the immune system and brings the body's natural yin/yang forces into harmony. Traditional Chinese medicine also depends upon such concepts as seasonal foods, food flavors, and even one's physical and mental constitution.

These concepts are based on the belief that food affects us because we are made up of both mind and matter. While every kind of food possesses a sustaining energy, each of us has special needs caused by our unique response to food and digestion. By ingesting foods that lack nutrition or substance—such as junk food, for example—we are unable to add to our store of *ch'i* energy. Worse, such unhealthy foods may actually weaken our *ch'i* and our immune system, thus making us vulnerable to fatigue and disease.

On the other hand, we can achieve optimal health and a spiritually enhanced diet by eating nutritionally potent foods that help us acquire greater *ch'i* energy. In *The Simple Path to Health*, acupuncturist and Chinese medicine teacher Kim Le writes that a basic diet, for example, requires that "at least 50% of each meal be made up of whole grains...About 20-30% of each meal should consist of locally grown organic vegetables...meals should also be composed of 5-10% soup." The remaining 10-25 percent consists of meat and seasonal fruits.

Viewed from the larger perspective of Eastern traditions and medicines, choosing a diet means encountering a sophisticated, holistic approach to health. Even the Buddha encouraged a holistic approach to health and longevity by promoting regular exercise, especially walking after meals, to aid digestion. And that was over two thousand years ago! Whether or not you accept the concept of *ch'i*, and other ideas mentioned here, the benefits we can gain by looking at our wholeness—as opposed to a formulaic one-size-fits-all approach—is well worth the effort.

Judaism—Food Suitable for Hallowing

For Judaism, a mindful or spiritual diet is one that hallows and adds meaning to life. In great part, this is the purpose of Jewish dietary laws, or *kashrut.* The laws guide Jews with regard to prayer and suitable foods. But even these laws—many of them detailed in the Bible's book of Leviticus—are not written in stone. They have adapted over time, just as our own mindful diet evolves the more that we learn, practice, and grow.

At the core of the Jewish mindful diet is a dilemma that has lasted centuries—for Jews as well as followers of other wisdom traditions: that of whether or not to eat the meat of sentient animals. Early in the book of Genesis, the ideal diet presented was simple and straightforward: "And God said, 'Behold, I have given you every plant yielding seed which is upon the face of all the earth, and every tree with seed in its fruit; you shall have them for food." Every fruit and vegetable was naturally *kosher*, or suitable and proper. Even today, there exist lineages of vegetarian Jews that continue to follow this simple law.

Later in Leviticus, however, there was an important change. Moses and Aaron were instructed by God to tell the Israelites that they could eat "animals that live on land," even detailing restrictions on which animals were acceptable. Samuel Dresner, in *The Jewish Dietary Laws*, describes this as "a divine compromise." While Adam was forbidden to eat meat in the Garden of Eden, Noah was permitted to satisfy his craving for meat under certain conditions.

Isn't this also a metaphor for humankind's predicament? If we could live in paradise—in the most pure, spiritual, and innocent state—then the taking of life would have no place. But since we inhabit earth—a place of desire, need, and human weakness—we compromise our ideal while at the same time honoring the life that we take. In return for our "divine compromise" we must show reverence through a personal sacrifice in terms of food, preparation, and prayer.

My own great-grandfather, Isaac, was a *shochet*—a religious man who ritually blesses and slaughters animals, thus making them kosher. Although I never met him, he was a full-bearded, quiet man, someone who faithfully observed the Sabbath and studied scripture; considering the difficult work he performed, such a regimen would certainly seem to be a necessity. Through the *shochet's* merciful techniques and blessings, kashrut acknowledges the harsh action of taking life that the unwelcome compromise of eating meat brings about.

Basically, kosher foods include all fruits and vegetables, cereals and grains, tame or domesticated herbivorous animals with cloven hoofs, fowl, fish with scales and fins, wine, milk, eggs, and cheese. Foods which are *treif*, or forbidden and nonkosher, include blood, carnivorous animals, animals hunted for sport, and shell fish. Pigs and rabbits are forbidden because they neither chew their own cud nor possess a cloven hoof. Also forbidden is the eating of meat and dairy products at the same meal; this is a dietary law stemming from the Bible's admonition not to cook a kid in its mother's milk.

In addition, kashrut contains regulations for keeping a kosher kitchen, such as maintaining separate dishes and utensils for meat and dairy products, removing all nonkosher food, and even using special methods for washing dishes. These laws—along with ritual washing of the hands, blessings, and other observances—teach a constant lesson about the hallowing of food and life.

Whereas Judaism is in part defined through its many food laws, Christianity is defined by its lack of dietary rules. Jesus himself made this point by declaring that outside agents, such as food, were not the cause of personal or spiritual defilement. Furthermore, his symbolic actions at The Last Supper—when he referred to bread as his flesh and wine as his blood—hinted at a new order that discarded the previous set of laws. In one stroke, all foods were declared "clean" and proper for consumption. Christianity thus set itself apart and declared itself distinct from Judaism. It was only in the sixteenth century that the Roman Catholic Church adopted a ban on eating meat on Friday—as a personal sacrifice. This restriction remained until the 1960s, when the Second Vatican Council relaxed many of its mandates.

Islam—Food According to God's Will

Islam follows dietary laws similar to Judaism's. Foods are classified as either *halal*, lawful, or *haram*, unlawful and forbidden. These rules help Muslims bring the blessings of nature, and God's desire that they eat properly, into daily life and daily practice. Basically, food is lawful and acceptable unless stated otherwise in the Qur'an or the Hadith. Generally, lawful foods include all marine animals, vegetables, fruits, grains, and dairy products. Meat is lawful only when slaughtered compassionately and in the name of Allah. Foods considered to be unlawful include alcohol, hallucinogens, and other substances that can intoxicate or harm the mind and body, or that can hinder our spiritual awareness.

Ultimately, Islam places the responsibility for choosing proper food on each individual. To choose properly, however, we need to be informed and knowledgeable. For example, while the Qur'an prohibits eating "the flesh of swine," it does not provide specific reasons why this is so. By leaving this prohibition undiscussed, Islam actively encourages the individual to seek out and analyze why some foods are forbidden while others are considered whole, pure, and beneficial.

As if anticipating the developments in synthetics, chemical fertilizers, food additives, pesticides, and perhaps, even food genetics, Muhammad in the Hadith says—as translated by Ahmad Sakr, Ph.D. in *A Muslim Guide to Food Ingredients*—"Halal is clear and Haram is clear; in between these two are certain things that are suspected...Anyone who gets involved in any of these suspected items, he may fall into the unlawful and the prohibition." Arabic uses two words to describe when the purity or ingredients of a food may be at issue. These are *mash-booh*, or "suspected," and *makrooh*, or "discouraged." If there is no written law regarding a food, or if someone simply doesn't know whether or not a food is lawful, then it is "suspect" and requires a decision based on one's own best judgment. "Discouraged" foods or habits are those known to be harmful to one's physical, mental, and spiritual health. These might include stimulants such as caffeine, and habits such as smoking.

Never before in history have we faced such a deluge of food choices. How do we cope with the onslaught of new food additives and processing techniques? If a sweetener or a synthetic fat is approved for use in food, does that mean we should go out and buy it? At what point is the thin line between a food and a drug crossed? If eating a food involves even a small risk, is that acceptable? We need to ask ourselves, as did Muhammad, if a food is suspect. There are enough whole, pure, and healthy foods available for us. Is the lure of lower calories or a lower fat content reason enough to take a risk with our health and our consciousness?

Personal Responsibility

It is a weekday. The bright morning sun peeks over a six-foot high, weathered red cinder-block wall at the monastery. Scattered on the ground I notice hundreds of long compass needles, maybe more—all perfectly aligned and pointing in the same direction. I have never seen anything like this. It seems they are pulled by some great magnetic force toward the rising sun. Then, looking closer, I realize that the compass needles are in reality the thin, long shadows cast by the tiniest of pebbles. Like shadow dancers, they stretch to greet the morning.

Life is like that, I think—for when all is said and done, our life choices scatter like a hundred thousand pebbles. Each acts as a compass that points us in a direction. The more we keep making spiritually aware choices, the stronger the compass reading becomes. Basically, it comes down to our personal responsibility to find out what is in the food we put into our body. How are our consciousness and physical health affected by hormones in meat, the bleaching of flour, the curing of meat, and the enrichment of cereals? If any of these are on our "suspect" list, what action do we take? These are not easy questions. Sometimes, even after diligent research there may be no clear answer. Given that we have the right expert advice—after all, we want to be sure we don't jeopardize our health—we use our own best judgment and inner self to guide us to a healthy, complete diet for mindful eating.

There was a long period in my life, for example, when a constant supply of diet sodas graced my refrigerator. Each quenched my thirst with the promise of "guiltless" pleasure. Although there were people who warned me about possible consequences, I continued buying and consuming these products and their artificial ingredients. Blind to any potential risk, all I could see was the calorie count on the label—as if that blotted out all else.

One day, however, I got a large envelope in the mail. It contained pages and pages of material sent to me by my mother—including research reports, personal stories, medical journal clippings, and newspaper articles on diet sodas. Whether the diet sodas I drank were injurious to me I do not really know. However, I can say that the more I read, the more they tripped into my personal "suspect" category.

There are many excellent books that offer enlightened approaches to food choices. Annemarie Colbin's *Food and Healing*, mentioned earlier, is one example of a compassionate and holistic approach to eating. It draws upon ancient Ayurvedic and Chinese philosophies, and includes information on healing through fasting, food combinations, and a balanced diet with the emphasis on fresh, unprocessed whole foods grown without chemicals or pesticides.

Being at the top of the food chain and depending on lower organisms may carry a degree of risk. As Andrew Weil writes, "One consequence of eating high on the food chain is that you take in much larger doses of toxins, because environmental toxins concentrate as you move up from level to level. The fat of domestic animals often contains high concentrations of toxins that exist in much lower concentrations in grains, for example."

The wisdom of ancient food laws shows that food has always been a tool for spiritual growth and healthy living. Whether following the precepts of an ancient tradition or creating traditions of our own, the choices we make regarding good and forbidden foods are with us every day and at every meal. The more we awaken to the idea of food as a healing medicine, the more attuned we will become to food's ultimate purpose and to finding a nourishing inner meal. This is all a part of the evolution of our mindful diet.

PRACTICE: DISCOVERING YOUR MINDFUL DIET

What is "suspect" is always subject to change. Still, we need to establish a personal guideline for foods we think are wholesome and healthy—and those that cross the line.

This does not mean we need to impose that guideline on others. A guideline can be thought of as a signpost that leads us down the road—until we reach the next sign. Use this practice as often as necessary, as a way to update your healthy food guidelines and stay informed.

Previously, you've discovered how to increase your awareness of habits and how to reflect on food's ultimate purpose. Now you have the opportunity to explore and shape your mindful diet. Remember that to eat in a consciously aware manner you need to make choices—even if they happen to be the wrong ones from time to time. The important thing is that you develop a useful guideline that will help make your decision-making process easier and your decisions better informed. This exercise is designed to do just that.

Take a sheet of paper and divide it into five columns. At the top of the first column write down the heading "Food Choices."

In the second and third columns, write down the headings "Evidence For" and "Evidence Against," respectively.

In the last two columns, add the headings "Recommended" and "Suspect."

After writing your present day eating choices in the first

column, see if you can determine the evidence for or against each listed item. If you have no evidence, simply leave that space blank. Once you have completed columns two and three, see if you can determine whether a food is "recommended" or "suspect."

In some cases, "suspect" means you need to do more research or investigation. In other cases, you may have all the evidence you need to decide that something is "suspect," and that you want to subtract it from your diet.

As you complete this list, keep in mind that you don't have to make rash decisions. You may not be sure how a food is affecting you. In some cases, you may decide that a "suspect" food is not harmful when eaten in moderation. Don't use this practice to become like the food police. Instead, think of it as gentle and wise advice from a dear friend who you love and respect.

Mostly, let yourself have fun with this practice. Go on the Internet and find out more about your food choices; check out interesting books and articles. You will most likely discover some fascinating and valuable information. Always, be mindful of the source.

As you add or subtract foods from your diet, pay special attention to how these new choices make you feel. Do they make you more energetic? Do they make you tired or drowsy? Or do they help you feel calm and alert? You may want to change only one food at a time in order to determine that food's effect. As with fasting, don't make major dietary changes without first consulting a physician or an appropriate health professional.

This exercise offers many advantages. It gives us the power and personal responsibility over what we eat. It builds confidence in our food selection. It gives us a barometer of how our mindful diet is evolving. Most importantly, it gives us the beginning of a plan for creating a beneficial and mindful diet.

14 – Nature's Connection

We did not come into this world.
We came out of it, like buds out of
branches and butterflies out of cocoons.
We are a natural product of this earth,
and if we turn out to be intelligent beings,
then it can only be because we are fruits
of an intelligent earth...

—Lyall Watson, *Gifts of Unknown Things*

An early rain has washed away the haze, and the air feels crisp and clean. For days now, I've been eyeing a three-acre commercial strawberry patch. When I've driven by it's usually empty, but this morning a number of pickers work the field. I drive onto a rutted dirt surface and park next to a covered strawberry stand. I ask the woman who works there if she can point me to the field's owner or foreman.

"What do you want?" she asks.

"I would like to pick strawberries," I say.

She stares at me for a moment, puzzled, then points to one of two men conversing near the stand. "Talk to him. His name is Camacho."

Camacho is a short, gray-haired man in his mid- to late fifties, wearing a plaid shirt. A gold neck chain glitters against his darkly tanned and weathered skin. After explaining that I am a writer and want to work an afternoon without pay, I half expect to be peppered with suspicious questions. But no, he tells me to report to the fore-man when the crew starts picking again at 2 o'clock that afternoon.

Back at the monastery I look for the proper clothing. A red sweatshirt to protect from the sun, and burgundy sweatpants—only too late do I realize that I have inadvertently dressed to resemble a strawberry. To make matters worse, my worn-out sneakers are no-where to be found and I have to wear my suede Hush Puppies. I quickly delude myself into thinking that picking a few strawberries will cause them no harm.

Arriving about ten minutes early I walk onto the field and see that a week of rain has left the ground soft and soggy. The foreman knows why I'm here, and he hands me a large cardboard box piled with empty pint containers and a rusted, broken-down three-wheeled pushcart. I fumble for a moment, not sure how the box and cart fit together. In Spanish, he calls on a teenager, maybe seventeen or eighteen years old, to help me. In unaccented English, the young man explains where to place the cart, how to stack the pints, which strawberries to pick, and which to avoid. He watches for a moment, then I'm on my own.

Feeling beneath and around each leafy green plant for the ripe red fruit is time-consuming. My technique for removing the strawberries from the stem needs work, and each one I bruise goes into my "seconds" bin. After five minutes I have less than a handful of good strawberries and a throbbing lower back. I look up at the row of strawberry plants before me; it stretches for several hundred feet. Determined to continue at all costs, I shift from a crouch onto my knees, flexing the Hush Puppies so the suede won't scrape the ground.

At root level, all the plants are covered with a plastic tarp. This protects them from certain bugs. The strawberry season lasts longer than that of many fruits—from early in the year through October. Because strawberries bruise easily, they have always been picked by hand. Finally, I discover how to bend the stem in a way that releases the fruit without harming it.

Every now and then a melody fills the air as someone sings a few words to a joyful, spirited song. I am reminded of stories I've heard about the growing of rice in Burma. In many villages, the planting and harvesting of the rice fields is a communal affair, complete with food, music, and song.

The singing around me lifts my spirits. I start to feel less self-conscious and even forget my back pain. Until now I hadn't noticed the crew. I look up briefly. About two dozen people work the field—both women and men, some much older than can easily do this work, or so I think. The women use bandannas to shade their heads and necks from the sun. All move quickly, filling their baskets in a fraction of the time it takes me. After an hour, I achingly straighten my spine and stand, my first box full. The young guide comes over and neatly rearranges the top layer, explaining that this is necessary for proper weighing and packaging.

The next box fills a little more quickly. At one point I notice a big yellow school bus that has paused for a stoplight. I look up at the school children, who look back at me. I wonder if they would like to be in the sunshine picking strawberries, too. Suddenly there is a hush of commotion and the young man calls to me, "The field is picked. We are done for the day." *So am I*, I muse to myself.

I strain to stand when something catches my eye. Glinting in the sun—if, indeed, fruit can glint—is the Hope Diamond of strawberries. The plump, perfectly shaped fruit is all for the taking, except that it's on the other side of a half-flooded irrigation channel. After a moment's contemplation I figure that if I edge along the dry side, it will be mine—a crowning finish to my almost full box.

I crouch, little by little sneaking up on the big red one. With each half step the ground grows softer beneath my feet. Finally, my prize is within reach. But as I stretch out my arm, the big red one just a fingertip away, my Hush Puppies slide down into the water.

I struggle to save my shoes, but the ankle-deep mud grips them with a *Titanic*-like determination. Undeterred, I grab the big red one while simultaneously trying to rescue my Hush Puppies. It requires an additional push of my hands on the ground to free my feet. Sopping wet from mud, I squish loudly with each step, looking and feeling very much like the now badly bruised big red one.

On the way back to the foreman, one of the crew—a middle-aged man—notices that I am a pint short a full box. He reaches in to his box, lifts out a pint of perfectly layered strawberries, and offers it to me. I shake my head, but he is insistent, and I am too tired and too touched by his kindness not to receive his heartfelt offer.

Before leaving, I stop at the stand to buy some strawberries for the monks. But when I walk up, the woman whom I had met earlier looks at me and asks a question that brings a smile to my lips:

"Would you like an aspirin?"

Sitting in my car moments later, I gather my thoughts. When we return to the fields from which life springs forth, I think, how can we not make the leap between mindful eating—indeed, any diet—and the Earth's ecological wellness?

A Diet for the Kingdom

I am reminded of an old tale about a wealthy and powerful king who, through circumstance, was separated from his only son. Eventually, the king found the boy. It turned out that he had no education, worked as a poor laborer, and had absolutely no idea who his father was.

The king, wanting to find out if the boy was worthy of his inheritance, arranged for him to work at the palace. Over time, the boy grew to take on more responsibility. When at last he reached manhood, the boy was brought to the king and told the truth—that he was in reality a prince to whom all the treasures of the kingdom will one day be entrusted.

This story illustrates how we may dwell in the kingdom of our all-knowing inner self without ever knowing it. This is also a metaphor for how we dwell in Earth's kingdom, often unaware that we are the princes and princesses to whom all its wondrous treasures are entrusted as a sacred responsibility.

Whether we connect with the Hindu and Buddhist concept of karma, the Judeo-Christian concept of stewardship, or the Pagan concept of a divine nature, the responsibility for Earth's care belongs to no one but ourselves. This is, after all, our home.

Treading the inner meal path brings an appreciation for the connectedness that ties together every remote corner of the Earth and the sky. Bound together as we are, our smallest action may exert a subtle ripple effect beyond our capacity to measure or comprehend. Certainly, the world has grown smaller, and effects of large-scale actions are now felt all across the globe. We are, as Native American mythology tells us, part of a sacred web:

> *All things are connected.*
> *Whatever befalls the earth,*
> *befalls the sons and daughters of the earth.*
> *Man did not weave the web of life;*
> *he is merely a strand in it.*
> *Whatever he does to the web,*
> *he does to himself.*

—Ted Perry (inspired by Chief Seattle), *how can one sell the air*

Unfortunately, it's the disasters that seem to accelerate our awareness of just how small and fragile our blue planet really is. Too often, the constant sounding of ecological alarm bells causes us to turn away in frustration and numbness. Global problems are just too massive and overwhelming for one person to deal with—whether it is pollution caused by a nuclear disaster, massive crop burning, or the loss of biodiversity in the rain forest and the ocean. After all, isn't it hard enough just to find the time to separate plastic, glass, and paper for recycling?

Here's the good news: in truth, your spiritual diet contains the capacity to impact the world—even if in a small way—simply by involving a change in the foods you eat. The Earth will do what it can. But as Native American Dan George points out, the job won't get done without our help:

Do not stop watering the corn while you count on the clouds to bring rain.

There is a danger in reducing the Earth—or ourselves, for that matter—to some kind of machine that can be worked ceaselessly and carelessly. Earth's resources are limited, its teeming life an interwoven and interdependent web upon which we depend. Ancient Buddhist thought tells us that the same degree of appreciation, importance, care, and respect we show our own mothers should also be accorded to our Earth. The Bible, too, tells us: "Six years you shall sow your field, and six years you shall prune your vineyard, and gather in its fruits; but in the seventh year there shall be a sabbath of solemn rest for the land, a sabbath to the Lord."

Though most of us aren't farmers, we can still find a way to provide a "rest for the land." When we practice fasting, for example, do we not also allow the Earth to fast by reducing the food demand, if ever so slightly? By observing the Sabbath or otherwise embracing a natural way of living even for a single day—such as reducing our energy and other consumption—do we not give the planet a much-needed sabbatical from our constant demands?

If you have doubts about your impact on this planet, spend a moment to think about the role butterflies play in the ecosystem. I still remember the day I happened upon thousands of orange-and-black monarchs floating through the air, like snowflakes, traveling on a migration extending as far as three thousand miles. According to Native American tradition, the butterfly represents balance and harmony. Butterflies are extremely sensitive to environmental changes, and when nature's harmony is upset they are among the first to be impacted. If that seems unimportant, consider that they pollinate the flowers of many plants. Just as the presence or ab-

sence of a butterfly can alter the course of nature, so can the diet of
one person impact and influence the Earth's resources and ecosystem.

Each of us possesses a small, self-contained ecosystem. This
temple of consciousness encompasses the relationship we have with
everything that goes in and out of our body and mind—including
what we eat, how we think, whom we associate with, how we
exercise, how we perform our work, and how we interact with the
large ecosystem of the Earth. In other words, nourishing the spirit
and nourishing the Earth go hand in hand. Knowing this, we may
want to ask ourselves, What diet benefits both the small and large
ecosystems at the same time? A diet that only partially fulfills the
needs of one, and not the other, may not in the long run be serving
either.

There are many ways to adjust and adapt your diet depending on where you live. Yet the one dietary constant contained in
wisdom traditions that can most impact the planet—other than adding whole, seasonal foods to your diet—is a near absence of meat.
While the basis for this choice relies upon the spiritual reasons discussed earlier, it also seems uncannily prescient and advantageous for
our present-day ecology—and maybe even your personal ecology.

There exists a mountain of information on how a meat-domi-
nated diet influences the larger ecosystem. Frances Moore Lappé, in
Diet for a Small Planet, details how cattle are a highly inefficient
form of protein. She demonstrates, for example, the cost of raising
cattle in terms of waste products (billions of tons a year), water
resources (twenty-five hundred gallons per pound of steak), and
the severe impact on soil erosion and ozone depletion.

The point here is not necessarily to stop eating beef, but to
become more aware of the consequences. Only you can seek the
path of your own inner meal wisdom. Whether or not you choose
to reduce your consumption of meat, eliminate it completely, or
even eat more is up to you.

The wisdom traditions—while they may present spiritual consequences of eating meat or other foods—generally make allowances for personal choice, special conditions, and the uniqueness

of each individual. What matters with mindful eating is that we are aware and awake enough—regarding our own patterns and habits, as well as the impact of our actions—to have freedom of choice. Annemarie Colbin writes in *Food and Healing* about the danger of "being stuck in *any* single, strict food ideology" or dogma. This may not only place our health in jeopardy, but also tell us about our habits and attachments.

If we are truly free to choose any food—or action, for that matter—then we have built up our will and strength to the point where we can resist that food, or action. This brings to mind the idea of nonresistance, of which Swami Prabhavananda in *The Spiritual Heritage of India* writes, "Nonresistance is recognized by all the great teachers as the highest virtue. The [Bhagavad] Gita also regards it as the highest virtue, but does not say that all people under all circumstances must practise it. On the contrary, it points out that for some it is necessary to learn to resist evil in order that by this means they may grow into a state in which they have the moral strength to endure it."

Ultimately, we are the ones who—through our awakened choice—determine which organic foods will be available at the market, and which additives and preservatives, if any, will go into our foods. In order to do this we need to go from being "smart" shoppers to "aware" shoppers. When you make a lifestyle change, even a small one, you also make a quiet, subtle impact on others—friends, family, and coworkers. Eating a spiritual diet balances both the small and large ecosystems—connected as they are—and reflects on the environment.

The Native American Chief Seattle expressed a deep love and reverence for the Earth in a well-known speech he gave in 1854. As written in his tender voice and plaintive words, may the spirits always be with us:

> *At night, when the streets of your cities and villages*
> *shall be silent, and you think them deserted,*
> *they will throng with the returning hosts*
> *that once filled and still love this beautiful land.*

PRACTICE: CONNECTING TO NATURE'S SOURCE

Like the roots of a tree that extend deeply into the ground, we too need to connect with nature's source in order to find our place within its sacred web. We need to know and feel these things: that much of the food in the supermarket originally grows from the ground, unpackaged and unprocessed, without artificial additives; that there are growing seasons for all things; that certain foods grow locally, while others are shipped or flown in from distant locales; that natural resources, energy, labor, and thought go into the planting and harvesting of our food; that all food requires water to grow and ripen.

And after knowing all this—deep in our being, heart, and inner self—we need to celebrate and bless the Earth that provides exactly what we require for life. Twentieth-century mystic and artist Walter Russell, in The Message of the Divine Iliad, *writes about discovering our purpose through being in balance with and connecting with nature's source:*

> *A man with a certain name lives at a certain address and thinks of himself as separate and apart from all Creation. A brook comes from the sea by way of the heavens. It seems to be a unit which is separated from everything else, but it is forever connected with the heavens and the sea. We do not see the connection between the heavens and the brook but they are, nevertheless, connected. Though we cannot* **see** *the connection, we can* **know** *it.*

This practice consists of two parts. The first part is, as Walter Russell writes, to *know* something as real even if it cannot be put into words. That "something" is to find our connection to the Earth that goes beyond our home address.

Find a quiet place to sit. Or, if you meditate, you can use the lotus position. Now, close your eyes and breathe gently.

Feel your "connection" to the chair or cushion on which you sit. Try to separate your "attachment" from your "connection." Perhaps you're attached to it because you picked it out because of its comfort. Or the color was pleasing. Or maybe it fit the decor of your room.

Your "connection" is your relationship to it. Try to feel this relationship. Now, expand outward to your living space, your "home address." Feel your connection to this place. Expand outward again, this time outside your home. Feel your relationship to the yard, the garden, or the neighboring birds, trees, homes, and neighbors. How interconnected are you with them? What is your relationship with them, if any? Allow yourself to feel whatever emotions this stirs in you—such as joy, happiness, or sadness. Don't analyze; simply allow yourself "to know." There are no right or wrong answers.

Expand once again, this time to a special place where you go to experience nature. It might be where you go camping. Or where you watch the sunset. It could be a park, a beach, an apple orchard, a gushing spring, a winding river, a canyon, a mountain, or a view of the stars and the moon. Hold the experience. Give yourself as much time as you need to feel this special place, its meaning, its relationship to you, and your sacred connection to it. Allow yourself to feel the awe, the beauty, and the joy of wonder that comes with a connection to nature's source. Remember this special place in your mind's eye, knowing that you can always return here and that you carry it with you in your heart at all times.

When you've finished, allow yourself to "contract" step by step until you've returned to your neighborhood, your home address, your home, your room, your chair.

The second part of this practice connects us to nature's source in a more real and practical way. Try to experience a connection with food and the soil. This can be done by spending a day at a farm or orchard, planting fruit tree, walking barefoot on the grass, starting an organic vegetable garden, or even going to the local farmers' market to get fresh seasonal foods. Try to learn the harvest seasons for the various foods you eat, especially those that are local, because they'll be freshest. If you have a family, make this a family activity; this is a fine way to develop a mutual dialogue about the purpose of nature and health.

The benefits of this practice are numerous. It lets us find renewed beauty and meaning in nature. We begin to sense the effects of our actions on the Earth, from diet to energy usage. It encourages us to learn more about the natural processes surrounding food and nutrition. It gives us an appreciation for the labor and effort that go into putting food into the market and onto our table. It provides an opportunity to bring our family together in a fun, meaningful, and purposeful way.

15 - A Personal Spiritual Ecology

*You would not expect much of your
radio if you abused it, nor can you
expect much conscious awareness if
you abuse your body. Your body is
receiver and transmitter...From it you
also broadcast that which is your idea
of Self. People know you by the broadcast
you give out from your sensed bodily
machine. You, yourself, tell all the world
whether you are jazz or symphony.*

—Walter Russell,
The Message of the Divine Illiad

How can we taste life's spiritual flavor? How do we augment our
spiritual capacity and strength in the midst of life's tribulations? And,
once having tasted and been nourished from this wellspring, how
can we continue to increase the flow of these pure waters? We can
begin by tasting each bite spiritually and mindfully. Here, we ini-
tiate the spirit into daily life. Here, we bring our spiritual self into
balance and harmony.

I remember a conversation I once had with a Benedictine monk who shared with me the effects that a major food change had on the monastic community in the 1960s. During that time, the reform movement of the Second Vatican Council modernized many of the restrictions on religious communities. As a result, some Benedictines gave up Gregorian chant—used since the Middle Ages—and substituted plainchant, which is now used with psalms and hymns. Others started eating meat. The consequences of these changes? Some people started getting sick. We know that even subtle modifications in diet can impact our health. But is the cause physical, spiritual, or both?

The physical and spiritual interact and cannot help but influence one another; the flow moves in both directions. At the moment of our birth, the two vital forces of breath and food combine to sustain life. The physical body transforms these into energy and spirit—with the potential to either energize or weaken us. The regulation of these two forces—through various forms of chanting, meditation, and mindful diet—alters our consciousness, enhances our spirit, and shapes our spiritual ecology, or ecospirituality. At the same time, it influences our physical and mental landscape.

The firsthand experiences of Gopi Krishna, chronicled in his book *Kundalini*, detail this two-way energy flow on the spiritual superhighway. When he was thirty-four years old, Gopi Krishna first tapped into and released his spiritual energy through a concentrated practice of Yoga. What he experienced was extraordinarily elating and harrowing—in both the physical and spiritual sense. As he relates in *Kundalini*, this newly found spiritual energy demanded a drastic change in his diet and even altered his sense of taste. After months of weakness, near fasting, and much experimentation with food, he discovered that "until the system grows accustomed to the flow of the radiant current, the one and the only preservative of life and sanity is diet in the right measure, correct combination, and at the proper intervals."

Unfortunately for us, Gopi Krishna did not provide a diary of his diet. Still, the wisdom traditions give us all the guidelines we need to bring our body and spirit into greater harmony. It is here, through the interaction between these two interdependent systems, that our personal ecospirituality takes shape. In this regard, Gopi Krishna concludes: "Almost all the methods in use from time immemorial for gaining visionary experience or supersensory perception—concentration, breathing, exercises, postures, prayer, fasting, asceticism and the like—affect both the organic frame and the mind. It is, therefore, but reasonable to suppose that any change brought about by their means in the sphere of thought must also be preceded by alterations in the chemistry of the body."

The ecospiritual part of us stretches far beyond our physical, sense-detecting limits. Yet it is always with us, cohabiting and balancing with our body, our life, and our world. As such, its health and care need to be of primary concern. A healthy and enlightened spiritual diet allows our body to receive a full measure of nourishment and energy from food. At the same time, it allows our spiritual capacity to expand and evolve.

The more frequently we practice mindful eating—or any spiritual practice—the deeper and stronger our spiritual capacity grows. You may not know it, but you are building a vision of your spiritual ecology at this very moment. We attain spiritual vision and strength by living in the present moment, learning all we can with humility and an open heart. We would do well to remember this prayer:

> God,
> Grant me the serenity to accept
> the things I cannot change,
> the courage to change the things I can,
> and the wisdom to know the difference.

Seven Steps to Strengthening Your Ecospirituality

First, tend to your spiritual ecology with great care and attention, for it is not much different from a garden. We may forget to feed our plants today, but we care enough about them to gently remind ourselves to make time for their watering tomorrow. The holiday of Tu B'Shavat is known as the Jewish Ecology Day. It's a time for planting trees and recognizing the sacred ecology of Earth that sustains us.

We, too, need to recognize that our spiritual ecology is rooted in our body and nourished by mindful eating. Make a commitment to follow a chosen spiritual discipline by which you cultivate this sacred space within. Add ritual blessing and prayer to your meal-time practice. This is how we attain spiritual power and strength.

The Buddha said if you want to accomplish something easily you need to be in the right place and environment, associate with the right people, eat the right food, and have the right attitude. Apply these ideas, and other good ones, to your spiritual ecology on a daily basis.

Second, serve others in love, and your ecospirituality will flour-ish. Use food as a pathway to reach and serve others. Feeding others the right foods bolsters their health, spiritual strength, and harmony. Know that your actions of kindness—be they small or large—truly matter and make a difference. What you give will return to you a thousand times in mysterious and often beautiful ways.

Third, listen deeply and meaningfully, and you will nourish your ecospirituality with tolerance, patience, and openness. This is a gift you give to yourself and others. By giving others a voice you help their story—and *your story*—come alive. Use your powers of mindfulness at mealtime to notice the needs of others. At the same time, be aware of the poles of giving and receiving—being open to both. When mealtime becomes sacred, you may find more and more opportunities to serve others as a mitzvah—from preparing meals and offering food to washing the dishes.

Fourth, be compassionate and moderate with your spiritual ecology. State your intent, then allow it to mature at its own pace. First we are children, then adolescents, then adults. Each phase must be experienced and lived before passing on to the next. When it's time to move on to the next stage, let go and move on. Practice some form of purifying and cleansing fasting as you let go of your patterns and habits, the old diet, and your hungry ghosts.

Your spiritual ecology right now is not the same as it was yesterday. Be gentle to yourself when you fall. Lift yourself up and start again. Learn to forgive, or at least try, and your spiritual ecology will return the favor.

Fifth, awaken to the subtleties, nuances, and spirits of the community called Earth, and your spiritual ecology will fill with joy and wisdom. Become aware of the often hidden lives of birds, insects, trees, flowers, foods, animals, and other living inhabitants of your world. Try to imagine the entire hierarchy of all living things. With our ability to interact with this planet—to make bread from wheat, wine from grapes, and houses from trees—we finish God's work.

When we walk the Earth without a sense of superiority, but with the sensibility of a humble guest, we honor Earth's ecology and our personal ecospirituality. Feel the difference of each breeze, or the power and energy surging from the ground. Aware and awake, you will begin to *know* and sense the world within a world within a world.

Sixth, find your blessings in things great and small, from the smallest grain of rice to the largest redwood tree. Find them in everyday things, like a glass of water. Find them in annoying things, like waiting in line at the grocery store. Find them in calming things, like silence and mindfulness. Find them in sweet things, like a shared meal. What's important is that you find them.

Seventh, accept what is known and what is unknown about your ideal diet, and your spiritual ecology will surrender to faith and uncertainty. Here, your potential remains unchained by expectation. Here, there exist no preconceived boundaries. Here, there resides the whole you, not just a part looking to lose weight or be fixed. Here, there dwells a new relationship to food. Here, it all gets done by letting go.

By creating our own vision of spiritual ecology we come full circle. The journey of discovery along the path of the inner meal is complete. Actually, it's only beginning, for now you enter the realm of art. Einstein once said, "The most beautiful experience we can have is the mysterious. It is the fundamental emotion which stands at the cradle of true art and true science."

May you set the table of your inner meal with artistry, love, and compassion. May you feel your interconnectedness in the sacred web through each food choice that you make. May you be free to choose the spiritual diet that satisfies your soul.

16 – Six Steps to Changing Food Habits

For the caravan of beings traveling
on the path of mundane existence
and starving for the meal of happiness,
it is the feast of happiness that satisfies
all sentient beings who have come as guests.

—Santideva, *A Guide to the Bodhisattva
Way of Life* (translated by Vesna Wallace
and B. Alan Wallace)

Having explored and experienced the power of mindful practices, it is now time for a well-earned feast. This feast is one of happiness and joy, and it stems from being able to activate your own mindful diet. Still, there are going to be cravings and temptations. There may be times when your newfound knowledge will be put to the test. But a misstep along the way doesn't mean your are lost; the path is still there. By using the six steps in this chapter as a guide, you will always be able to find your way home to your mindful diet.

Over the past twenty years, disordered eating has become epidemic in the United States. It is estimated that as many as 10 million women suffer from anorexia nervosa, bulimia nervosa, and binge eating disorder. The number of men being treated for these problems is also increasing. In our body-image conscious world, there are other forms of disordered eating that are less severe and non-pathological, but just as troublesome—such as holiday overeating, the never-ending diet, and the 10-minute corporate cubicle meal. Many of our ingrained habits are not only personal, but cultural. How do we go about changing them?

It may be helpful to first ask, What will a change in food habits mean? For example, does it mean that you will never again overeat on Thanksgiving, never have another food craving, or never eat another meal too quickly? That might be nice, but is it realistic?

Understanding Acceptance, Commitment, and Skill

There is more than one way to understand change. Many of us are familiar with the mechanical, or replacement, view of change. From this perspective, we change things by eliminating whatever is mechanically broken or undesirable and replacing it with something new. This works when our car breaks down, and we replace the broken parts or buy a car that comes with a warranty. Some medical treatments also successfully follow this model by replacing body joints and even hearts. But can we truly have a warranty on our food choices? The problem with a mechanical and replacement view of change is that it forces us into all-or-none thinking. We must completely fix ourselves—and our desires—in order to be good, perfect, and worthwhile; if we cannot fix ourselves, then we are broken, defective, and unworthy.

A second perspective on change stresses the importance of acceptance, commitment, and skill. This approach is more forgiving because it allows space for making wrong turns. It acknowledges that we need not be perfect in our quest to have more healthful eating habits. In fact, it encourages us to accept the fact that stress, food static, and emotional turbulence may increase our tendency to fall back on established patterns. But take heart—this is only a tendency, not a permanent edict written in stone.

If we make a commitment to learn the skills that can help us weather difficult emotional storms, then we will have greater success at making changes. This more gentle perspective recognizes that change doesn't happen all at once, but in baby steps that we can take in this moment. For example, I have had some workshop participants who told me that they couldn't practice mindful breathing for five minutes a day. When I asked if they could practice for thirty seconds a day, they agreed. To me, any effort is still change, still a success. Change does not have to be scary if it beats with a heart of acceptance, commitment, and skill.

Six Steps to Changing Food Habits

Eating is not a race, but a place to find grace. What matters most is that you focus on realistic changes as you practice and experience each step.

Step One: Acknowledge Your Habits. We need to see the reality of our habits before we can step onto the path of change. Fortunately, this kind of acknowledgment is nonjudgmental and nonblaming. It doesn't label us with names or call us a failure. It doesn't shackle us with feelings of shame or guilt. The key is to let your acknowledgment come from the mindful and liberating awareness of what is, without adornment or exaggeration. Simply *what is.* Nothing more or less. What a wonderful starting point.

From here we can bring compassion—not only for ourselves, but for others who struggle with food issues. Rather than interpret our struggle as a weakness, we can realize that every wise person has grown through adversity. We can gain hope by understanding that acknowledgment is a salve that starts the healing process. Each earthly lesson is just what we require at this exact moment. Consider, for example, how a butterfly's struggle to escape from its cocoon gives it the strength it needs to fly. Likewise, our awareness and acknowledgment empower us to alter the course of our habits.

If you are not sure about the reality of your habits, you can always monitor them for yourself on a sheet of paper. Or enlist the constructive feedback of others. Remember that you are acting as a detective searching for clues. Don't be a judge and jury.

Step Two: Accept and Forgive Yourself and Others. Acceptance and forgiveness are like purifying waters that carry us gently and tenderly into the river of change. Acceptance means not viewing ourselves as defective or less than whole. With acceptance, we just *are*, which may be unskillful at times—but that does not mean that we can't become more skillful. When we fully and compassionately accept our history and our tendencies, we are more ready to forgive ourselves if we happen to step off the path.

Forgiveness comes in many colors. We can forgive those who have hurt us, those who we have hurt, and even ourselves—for self-inflicted hurt. We need to release all these kinds of hurt. If you think about it, if we do not forgive, how can we expect the grace of being forgiven? Forgiveness is a two-way street. In *The Art of Forgiveness, Lovingkindness, and Peace*, Jack Kornfield includes wisdom from many sources, including these words from Ajahn Chah:

> *If you let go a little,*
> *you will have a little happiness.*
> *If you let go a lot*
> *you will have a lot of happiness.*
> *If you let go completely*
> *you will be free.*

How do we let go of our anger, our bitterness, and our regret? This is not always easy. Bear in mind that forgiving doesn't mean forgetting. Even if we can't forgive a lot, maybe we can forgive a little. If forgiving others seems too painful, it may help to ask these questions: Who among us has never been hurt? Haven't we all suffered in some way? With forgiveness we can cultivate inner peace and give ourselves the space to change.

Step Three: Make a Vow to Change. Have you ever made a New Year's resolution to lose weight, only to forget about it later?

Next time, instead of making a resolution, you may want to consider taking a vow. Actually, there is quite a difference between the two. A vow is a formalized resolution, or commitment, to do something. Vows serve several important purposes: they commit us to a more formal discipline; they challenge us to stay on our path; they help guard us against stepping off the path. Often, vows are taken in public, like wedding vows. Sometimes they are performed in the presence of a minister, rabbi, or other spiritual guide. This makes us accountable and helps us feel the substance of a vow. Whether you decide to create a private or public vow, do what you can to make the ceremony meaningful.

Vows are not magic pills that make issues disappear. But when taken seriously, your vow to change will serve as a knowing guide. You might, for example, decide to eat mindfully once a day or once a week. This could be a full meal, or it could be a snack. Or you might choose to eat one healthy meal a week. Whatever you decide, focus on letting your vow lead you toward small and achievable steps.

Spend some time thinking about how to structure your vow. Write it down as clearly as possible. Include those ways you can support it, either through a morning prayer or some means of repeating it. When you find yourself succeeding, don't be in a big hurry to change your vow. Let it settle in for a few weeks. Then, when you feel you're ready for another small step, revise it. Remember to do so in a mindful, sacred, and spiritual way.

Step Four: Create a New, More Skillful Karma. While our karma may be in the refrigerator, that is not the only place it resides. We need to think about other factors that influence our food choices. These factors fall into three basic categories: backup skills, lifestyle skills, and thinking skills.

Backup skills are easy to understand. They are how we protect ourselves in case of emergency, such as driving with a spare tire in the trunk of the car or having a fire extinguisher in the house. Likewise, how do you protect yourself against potential food emergencies? Do you have a backup plan for those times that you only have a few minutes to eat while at work or on the run? Do you have a backup plan in your refrigerator at this very moment? If all you have is a box of donuts or a bowl of candy at home, then you might as well be driving on a flat tire, with no spare in the trunk.

You can create backup skills by first identifying those times, places, and situations that lead to emergency eating. Next, take the steps necessary to ensure that some healthy foods will be available for you during any situation—emergency or otherwise. In general, broaden the food choices that are within your reach. This may mean preparing little bags of healthy snacks that you can carry in your purse or briefcase. Consider, too, that a backup plan could include having someone to talk to when you are feeling upset or lonely. Don't put limitations on your backup skills. You are showing that you are prepared and care enough to create a new food karma.

The next category, lifestyle skills, are those actions that support your overall well-being on a daily basis. These include such basics as practicing mindful and relaxed breathing, getting enough sleep and exercise, eating nutritious foods, and finding pleasure. By pleasure I mean noting anything that brings you joy. This can include taking a short walk, enjoying nature, and talking with someone you like. Feeling good motivates us, and pleasure can be found in almost any activity—even in mindfully washing the dishes!

If these practices are overlooked, you may diminish your ability to change. Why is this so? For example, I have a very close friend who tried for several years to quit smoking. She was unsuccessful until she started making choices that were incompatible with her smoking habit. Once she began a regimen that included getting enough exercise, sleep, and healthy foods, she experienced herself in a new way—as someone living a healthy lifestyle. Rather than trying to eliminate a habit that probably felt good on some level, she added new behaviors that made her feel even better as a whole person.

You can begin by assessing your current lifestyle skills. How much sleep do you get each night? Does the Food Inventory practice in chapter 2 indicate the need for a nutritional adjustment? Have you incorporated mindful breathing into your daily life as a way to reduce stress? How much exercise do you get weekly? Are you enjoying something each day?

Now devise a plan that helps you bring these practices into your life in small ways. For example, if you are getting less than eight hours of sleep a night, you might try creating a calming night-time ritual. This could include mindful breathing, listening to soothing music, and sipping chamomile tea or warm milk. When adjusting your nutrition, it is advisable to seek the guidance of a doctor or dietitian.

One more category affecting food choices is that of thinking skills. Here, you can begin by examining thoughts with nonjudgmental, bare awareness—as covered in chapter 3. The point here is not to completely eliminate narrow and unskillful thoughts. Nor is it to find fault. Rather, it's about cultivating tolerance and compassion for ourselves by broadening our consistently one-sided thoughts and ideas. Just as every magnet has two opposing magnetic poles, we can have opposing views and still be a whole person.

As you do this, it may help to remember that you can simply observe your thoughts without being attached to them or letting them define who you are. Don't be surprised if you experience many different kinds of thinking patterns. For example, a thought habit that states "I'll never lose any weight" or "I'll always overeat," typifies all-or-none thinking. Another limiting pattern is to blame yourself: "It's my fault this is happening." Yet another one is misery-making: "This is going to turn out for the worst, it can't work." Then there is emotional overload: "I am so upset and frustrated that I want to give up." Also, let's not forget guilty thinking, which sounds like this: "I shouldn't have eaten that extra helping," or "I knew I would go off my plan."

Now, since there are two sides to every idea, imagine how you could broaden a limiting statement. Suppose your thought is "I'll never be able to eat right." Is it really true? What evidence do you have for a broader, more beneficial view? You could, for example, try to think of even *one* healthy food that you have eaten recently. Once your limiting idea becomes more balanced, write it down. This might be, "Come to think of it, I have eaten some good foods when I'm not stressed out." Next, practice saying this new thought out loud. Rehearse these broader thoughts as often as you can. It takes time to develop more open and skillful thinking patterns.

Just like the wise and patient gardener, you can know that having some weeds won't stop you from planting new seeds. One day your seeds will naturally grow and flower into a beautiful garden.

Step Five: Practice Mindfulness. Someone once asked me if problem solving was a mindful activity. When you about it, there isn't anything that you can't be mindful about. Whether you are walking, reading, being creative, eating, exercising, or thinking, you can apply mindfulness to your mental and physical activities. You can, for example, be mindful of your body position when you are sitting, standing, or exercising. Be mindful of the tension in your neck and shoulders. How is your spine positioned? Usually, we move our body when there is some discomfort. The next time you sit in a chair for an extended length of time, try to become aware of fatigue. This will help you move intentionally, with mindfulness.

As mindfulness becomes a greater part of your life, you will feel each moment as something precious, not to be wasted. This, too, is part of mindful eating.

Step Six: Invite the Sacred into Your Meals. Use the mindful seasonings of ritual blessings, Lectio, statio, the tea ceremony principles, moderate and compassionate fasting, precepts, simplicity, prayer, the Sabbath, communion, and others as often as you can. Adapt them, if necessary, for your own family and work situation. You may even decide to follow the spiritual meal guidelines that are in this book. Above all, be creative and trust your instincts. With mindfulness, you will find a way to make food a healthy and sacred part of life.

17 – Mindfulness...

As I near the end of my journey into the art of the inner meal I have returned to my home near the beach. A passing winter storm has left the sand compact and saturated beneath my feet. A rainbow of perfectly constructed miniature shells, once a sea creature's home, scatter along the beach. Two surfers in black wet suits, resembling seals from a distance, float in the foamy green surf.

A lone heron glides and suddenly dives headfirst into the froth. Moments after swallowing a fish whole, the bird scuttles along the surface for a few moments. Powerful flaps loft it skyward near the front edge of a massive wave. The curling water lifts the surfers and catapults them forward. The wave crests mightily, finally breaking under its own weight. The waters subside and the surfers reappear. The heron, in the distance now, merges with the grey sky...

Bibliography and Further Reading

Aggañña Sutta [Discourse on Genesis], From the Pathika Vagga Pali,
    Suttanta Pitaka, also known as the 3rd Book, 2nd Basket
Armstrong, Karen, *A History of God* Ballantine Books, 1993, NY
_____, *Muhammad* HarperCollins, 1993, New York
Bakhtiar, Laleh, *Sufi Expressions of the Mystic Quest* Thames and
    Hudson, 1976, New York
Berry, Rynn, *Famous Vegetarians & Their Favorite Recipes*
    Pythagorean Publishers, 1996, New York
Bryant, Page, *Native American Mythology* HarperCollins, 1991, NY
Buber, Martin, *I and Thou* Charles Scribner's Sons, 1970, New York
Buswell, Robert Jr., *The Zen Monastic Experience* Princeton, 1992,
    NY
Byrom, Thomas, *Dhammapada: The Sayings of the Buddha*
    Shambhala, 1993, Boston & London
Campbell, Dawn L., *The Tea Book* Pelican Books, 1995, Louisiana
de Vogüé, Adalbert, *To Love Fasting* Saint Bede's Publications, 1988,
    Petersham, MA
Cheewa, James, *Catch the Whisper of the Wind* Health Communica-
    tions, Inc. 1995, Deerfield Beach, FL
Chittister, Joan, *Wisdom Distilled from the Daily* HarperCollins, 1989,
    New York
Cleary, Thomas, *Living a Good Life* Random House, 1997, New York
_____, ed. *The Essential Confucius* HarperCollins, 1992, New York
_____, *The Essential Koran* HarperCollins, 1993, New York
Cleary, Thomas, *Living a Good Life* Random House, 1997, New York
Colbin, Annemarie, *Food and Healing* Ballantine Books,1996, NY
Cooper, J. C., *The Dictionary of Festivals* Thorsons, 1995, London
Cooper, John, *Eat and Be Satisfied* Jason Aronson Inc, 1993, New
    Jersey & London
Curry, Brother Rick, *The Secrets of Jesuit Breadmaking*
    HarperCollins, 1995, New York
De Silva, Cara ed. *In Memory's Kitchen* Translated by Bianca Steiner

Brown, Jason Aronson Inc., 1996, New Jersey and London

Dogen and Uchiyama, *From the Zen Kitchen to Enlightenment* Weatherhill, Inc., 1983, New York

Dresner, Samuel H., and Siegel, Seymour, *The Jewish Dietary Laws* The Rabbinical Assembly of America and United Synagogue Commission on Jewish Education, 1982, New York

Fingarette, Herbert, *Confucius—the Secular as Sacred* Harper Torchbooks, 1992, New York

Fiszar, Louise, & Ferrary, Jeannette, *Jewish Holiday Feasts* Chronicle Books, 1995, San Francisco, CA

Fox, Rabbi Karen L., and Miller, Phyllis, *Seasons for Celebration* Perigee Books, 1976, New York

Frank, Karl Suso, *With Greater Liberty* Cistercian Publication, 1993, Kalamazoo, MI

Fremantle, Francesca, & Trungpa, Chogyam, *The Tibetan Book of the Dead* Shambhala, 1987, Boston, MA

Glassman, Bernard, & Fields, Rick, *Instructions to the Cook* Bell Tower, 1996, Boston & London

Gordis, Daniel, *God was not in the Fire* Touchstone, 1995, New York

Hanh, Thich Nhat, *Our Appointment with Life* Parallax, 1990, Berkeley, CA

Harlow, Rabbi Jules editor and translations, *Siddur Sim Shalom, Prayerbook for Shabbat, Festivals, and Weekdays* The Rabbinical Assembly & The United Synagogue of Conservative Judaism, 1985, New York

Harvey, Andrew, *The Essential Mystics* HarperCollins, 1996, NY

Heinerman, John, *Heinerman's Encyclopedia of Anti-Aging Remedies* Prentice Hall ,1996, NJ

Heschel, Abraham Joshua, *The Sabbath* The Noonday Press, 1996, New York

Hill, Thelma, *Too Deep For Words* Paulist Press, 1988, NJ

Holy Bible, The Revised Standard Version

NIV Study Bible New International Version

Khan, Inayat, *Notes From The Unstruck Music from The Gayan of Inayat Khan* Message Publications, 1985, Tucson, Arizona

Kalechofsky, Roberta, & Rasiel, Rosa, *The Jewish Vegetarian Year Cookbook* Micah,1997, New York

Kamenetz, Rodger, *The Jew in the Lotus* HarperCollins, 1994, NY

Keating, Thomas, *Open Mind, Open Heart* Continuum, 1986, NY

Kertzar, Rabbi Morris, *What is a Jew?* Touchstone, 1996, New York

Krishna, Gopi, *Kundalini* Random House, 1997, New York

Kornfield, Jack, *A Path with Heart* Bantam, 1993, NY & London

_____, *Teachings of The Buddha* Shambhala, 1996, Boston & London

_____, *The Art of Forgiveness, Lovingkindness, and Peace* Bantam, 2002, New York & London

Lappé, Frances Moore, *Diet for a Small Planet* Random House, 1971,
    New York
Lao Tzu, translation: Blakney, R.B., *The Way of Life* Penguin Books,
    1983, New York
Le, Kim, *The Simple Path to Health* Rudra Press, 1986, Portland, OR
Johanson, Greg, & Kurtz, Ron, *Grace Unfolding* Bell Tower, 1991,
    New York
Mahasi, Sayadaw, *Fundamentals of Vipassana Meditation*
    Dhammachakka Meditation Center, 1991, Berkeley, CA
Maitreya, Balangoda Ananda, *The Dhammapada* Parallax Press,
    1995, CA
Mascaró, Juan, *Bhagavad Gita* Penguin Books, 1962, New York &
    London
_____, *The Upanishads* Penguin Books, 1965, New York & London
McClure, Joy, & Layne, Kendall, *Cooking for Consciousness* Nucleus
    Publications, 1993, Willow Springs, MO
Neihardt, John, *Black Elk Speaks* University of Nebraska Press, 1995,
    Lincoln & London
Norris, Kathleen, *The Psalms* Riverhead Books 1997, New York
Novak, Philip, *The World's Wisdom* HarperCollins, 1995, New York
Okakura, Kakuzo, *The Book of Tea* Shambhala, 1993, Boston &
    London
Panati, Charles, *Sacred Origins of Profound Things* Penguin Books,
    1996, New York
Prabhavananda, Swami, *The Spiritual Heritage of India* Vedanta
    Press, 1963, New York
Prabhavananda, Swami, & Isherwood, Christopher, *The Song of God:
    Bhagavad-Gita* Mentor Books, 1972, CA
_____, *Crest-Jewel of Discrimination* Hollywood, CA: Vedanta Press,
    1947
Prayers & Praises in the Celtic Tradition Templegate Publishers, 1986,
    London
Reinhart, Brother Peter, *Brother Juniper's Bread Book* Addison
    Wesley, 1991, Reading, MA
Roszak, Theodore, & Gomes, Mary, & Kanner, Allen, *Ecopsychology*
    Sierra Club Books, 1995, CA
Rowling, Marjorie, *Life in Medieval Times* Perigee Books, 1976, NY
Rule of St. Benedict In English, The The Liturgical Press, 1982,
    Collegeville, Minnesota
Russell, Walter, *Message of the Divine Iliad, The* The University of
    Science and Philosophy, 1971, Swannanoa, Waynesboro,
    Virginia
Ryan, M. J. Editor, *A Grateful Heart* Conari Press, 1994, Berkeley, CA
Sakr, Ahmad H., *Fasting Regulation and Practices* Foundation for
    Islamic Knowledge, 1991, Illinois

_____, *A Muslim Guide to Food Ingredients* Foundation for Islamic Knowledge, 1993, Illinois

_____, *Understanding Halal Foods* Foundation for Islamic Knowledge, 1996, Illinois

Santideva, *A Guide to the Bodhisattva Way of life*, translated by Vesna Wallace and B. Alan Wallace, Snow Lion, 1997, New York

Scott, David, & Doubleday, Tony, *The Elements of Zen* Barnes & Noble, 1997, New York

Seattle, Chief, *How Can One Sell The Air?* The Book Publishing Co., 1992, Summertown, TN

Sen XV, Soshitsu, *Tea Life, Tea Mind* Weatherhill, Inc., 1995, New York & Tokyo

Shah, Idries, *The Way of The Sufi* Dutton, 1968, New York

Shu'aib, Tajuddin, *The Prescribed Prayer Made Simple* Da'awah Enterprises International, 1983, CA

Silananda, Venerable U, *Four Foundations of Mindfulness* Wisdom Publications, 1990, MA

Smith, Huston, *Forgotten Truth* HarperCollins, 1976, New York

_____, *The World's Religions* HarperCollins, 1991, New York

Spiller, Gene, & Hubbard, Rowena, *Nutrition Secrets of the Ancients* Prima Publishing, 1995, CA

Spiritual Diary Self-Realization Fellowship, 1996, Los Angeles

Tanakh: Holy Scriptures, The The Jewish Publication Society, 1985, Philadelphia & Jerusalem

Teachings of Sri Ramakrishna Advaita Ashrama, 1994, Mayavati, Pithoragarh, Himalayas

Tun, Sao Hmat M., *Handbook of Buddhist Recitation* Dhammikarama [Burmese] Buddhist Temple, Malaysia

Verma, Vinod Dr., *Ayurveda for Life* Samuel Weiser, Inc., 1997, New York

Versluis Arthur, *Sacred Earth* Inner Traditions International, 1992, Rochester, Vermont

Vivekananda, Swami, *Practical Vedanta* Advaita Ashrama, 1995, Calcutta

Walker Bynum, Caroline, *Holy Feast and Holy Fast* University of California Press, 1987, CA

Walshe, John G., & Warrier, Shrikala, *Dates and Meanings of Religious and Other Festivals*, Foulsham, 1997, London & NY & Toronto & Sydney

Watson, Lyall, *Gifts of Unknown Things*, Bantam Books, 1978, NY

Weil, Andrew, *Spontaneous Healing* Fawcett Columbine,1995, NY

Williamson, Marianne, *Illuminata* Berkeley Publishing Group, 1994, New York

Yogananda, Paramahansa, *God Talks With Arjuna: The Bhagavad Gita* Self-Realization Fellowship, 1995, Los Angeles

Index